The Genesis of Jake

The Genesis of Jake

A Baby Story

Monica Eggen

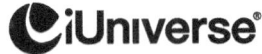

THE GENESIS OF JAKE
A BABY STORY

iUniverse books may be ordered through booksellers or by contacting:

iUniverse
1663 Liberty Drive
Bloomington, IN 47403
www.iuniverse.com
1-800-Authors (1-800-288-4677)

Because of the dynamic nature of the Internet, any web addresses or links contained in this book may have changed since publication and may no longer be valid. The views expressed in this work are solely those of the author and do not necessarily reflect the views of the publisher, and the publisher hereby disclaims any responsibility for them.

Any people depicted in stock imagery provided by Getty Images are models, and such images are being used for illustrative purposes only. Certain stock imagery © Getty Images.

"Tender is the Night", 1985, courtesy of Asylum Records. Written by Jackson Browne, Russell Kunkel & Danny Kortchmar.

ISBN: 978-0-5952-8876-2 (sc)
ISBN: 978-0-5956-5921-0 (hc)
ISBN: 978-0-5957-4892-1 (e)

Print information available on the last page.

iUniverse rev. date: 01/23/2020

for Scott

Tender is the night...
When you hold your baby tight—
Tender are the motions,
Tender is the night.

—*Jackson Browne*

Contents

Part I:
Before Jake Arrives

February 25, 1997: Scott and Monica meet for the first time. First date at Red Robin in Mesa, Arizona. Within weeks we both realize this is something very special. We spend most every day together from this day forward; eventually, six months into our engagement, we move in together.

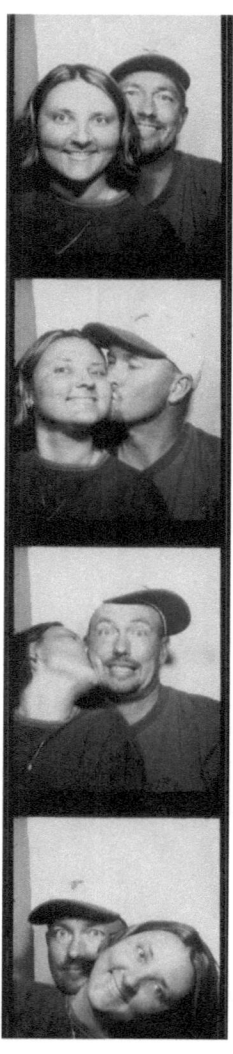

November 18, 2000: Monica, 31, and Scott, 33, wed in a beautiful outdoor ceremony at Tovrea Mansion in Phoenix, in front of 150 of our closest friends, family and colleagues. We are told by many that the reception is fun and memorable. We begin our married life in unpredictable fashion: exit via helicopter into the Phoenix night sky. Tomorrow, we're off to enjoy Kauai.

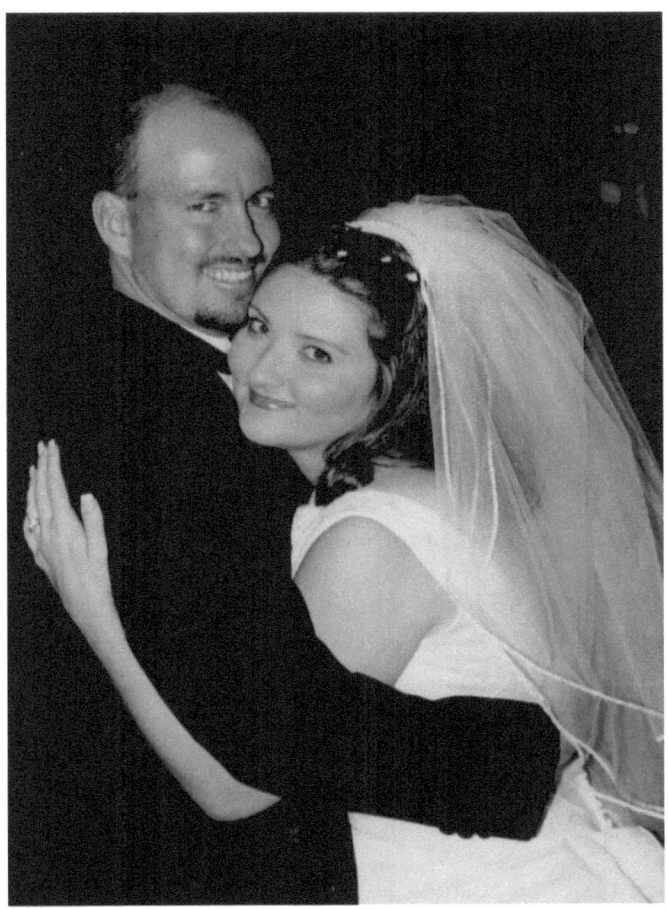

May 27, 2001: Six months into this marriage, Monica goes off the pill. We recognize that we're not getting any younger and we're ready to try to make an addition to "Team Eggen"! Well, we might not be totally ready to be parents, but we're as ready as we're gonna get! We feel good about our choice.

June 22: We're off to the races. Monica gets her period on the 30th day. Getting serious about this business now. I buy a basal thermometer to try to predict ovulation.

July 8: Tired of trying to take my temperature at the exact same time of day, "immediately upon awakening from sleep in the morning before doing anything else." Too stressful to try to go back to sleep when I wake up early.

July 21: Period #2 since going off the pill, now at 30-day cycle, if you count day one as first day of period. It should be pretty easy to predict ovulation at 14 days before period. Interesting that sperm can live for up to 72 hours, but eggs will dissolve within 24 hours.

August 11: Small amount of spotting—could this be from implanting? Feeling hopeful about the possibility.

August 18: 29th day since my last period started. Getting very antsy. Take a pregnancy test at 7 a.m. Not pregnant.

August 19: Period #3 starts since going off the pill, remaining fairly consistent at 30-day cycle. I feel okay about it because I appreciate having another month to again try to lose five pounds before I get pregnant.

September 6: I've had clear discharge for 3 days. One day is typical during ovulation for me, so this is unusual. What does it mean?

September 11: On a business trip, I spend this heartbreaking day with a coworker. I miss Scott so much. "Our hearts are at half-mast."

September 14: Janell and I arrive home after a long drive from Michigan via Illinois. I missed Scott's 34th birthday and the Laser Tag surprise party I planned.

September 17: Period due today if 30-day cycle consistent.

September 18: Pregnancy test negative. Period starts in the evening, on the 31st day of cycle.

October 17: 30th day of next cycle. Nothing.

October 18: 31st day of cycle. Nothing.

October 19: Pregnancy test negative. I'm so disappointed.

October 21: Still nothing. There's still hope this month. Nerve-racking.

October 22: Monday morning. It's time to take another test. The pregnancy hormone levels would have increased by now. Our pregnancy test is... **POSITIVE! WOW!!!!!!!!!!!!!** We are SO excited, but a little nervous. What are we getting ourselves into...? We conceived our baby on October 3 or 4, 2001. We are the only two people that know our titillating secret, just for one night. What a fabulous secret.

October 23: Scott and I have talked about not telling people yet. And for sure only family for the first trimester. I tell my mom and sister, Heidi, today, after having promised to tell them immediately upon knowing I was pregnant. On the pregnancy.about.com website, I calculate our due date as June 25, 2002.

October 25: I tell my dad and my boss that we are expecting.

October 26: We are three weeks from conception, "five weeks" pregnant since we learn that it actually starts from the last period.

October 27: The Diamondbacks win Game 1 of the World Series. We tell Mary, Doug, Duane, Mackenzie and Jason our news, which manages to outshine the game! Mary later today tells Holly.

October 28: We go to Game 2. Baby, too. We tell Sean the news.

October 29: This week we tell Nick, Brad and Ed (he saw a congratulations card on our bookshelf so the secret was out).

November 2: We are four weeks from conception and "six weeks" pregnant. I've noticed I have many of the "symptoms" now: I'm very sensitive to smells (especially smokers coming back inside after smoking), tired (more than usual, especially in the evenings after work), gassy/crampy (with some diarrhea), a little queasy but no morning sickness yet, and I'm more frequently feeling irritated.

November 3: Blame it on the pregnancy? Just two years into my lease, I trade in my VW Passat and lease a Mazda Tribute, with Scott out of town. I did forewarn him, though. I've wanted one for awhile, but I'm thinking now about loading and unloading a car seat. The Tribute has a 5 star crash test rating, which doesn't hurt. I so loved my Passat, but really want to sit up higher. I need to keep the Tribute for at least 4 years to break even with payoff/trade-in value.

November 4: Our beloved Diamondbacks win the World Series! Schilling/Johnson co-MVPs...I'm very excited to go to the doctor! I have to wait until November 27th. It's weird to not have gone yet, but both OB/GYNs I called said no openings are available until then and that it's "normal" not to be seen until the 8th week or so. My book says you're seen right away. I may call my Primary Care Physician.

November 6: I visit my PCP just to touch base with a doctor.

November 7: Fasting blood test today. I have to wait to eat breakfast until after my blood is drawn. Results came out "great"—oh, and positive for pregnancy, too. It's nice to have an official confirmation.

November 13: We are now eight weeks along. My pregnancy this week: I'm still very tired (plus being busy at work is not helping); I have VERY sore and sensitive breasts; my pants don't fit unless they have elastic waists; I'm not enjoying many smells, including my new car smell, the manure (we are seeding for winter grass this week) and the smell of new carpet and chemicals in OmniMount's board room; I'm sometimes starving, but trying to eat healthy; I'm very thirsty and drinking lots of water (it wasn't hard to give up Diet Coke after the first week), and I'm making lots of trips to the potty to pee!

November 17: It's Saturday, but I work 9 a.m.—1:30 p.m. then nap. Scott and I go to the Marquesa for our anniversary dinner. It's a long evening, with dinner lasting from 7:30—10 p.m. We take a very nice walk around the Scottsdale Princess after dinner.

November 18: Our one-year wedding anniversary—we work for two hours on our Hawaii scrapbook, which is lookin' good! It would be nice to finish it before the baby arrives (unlikely?).

November 25: Scott finished reading *Fellowship of the Ring* to me. He also read me *The Hobbit* this year. It's been really fun.

November 27: We are at ten weeks and have our first OB visit. Scott accompanies me to Dr. McN.'s office for our 9:10 a.m. appointment. I pay a $10 copay and **that's it** for all my prenatal visits! Scott and I see our baby for the first time at 10:30 a.m. today! (Vaginal wand ultrasound—amazing—although it looked strange, it wasn't uncomfortable like I thought it might be) We see its little beating heart! Scott: "I can't believe we actually saw little arms and the heart. This is awesome!"

November 29: I still haven't told anyone at work and it's still a secret. However, today Gregory guesses about the baby when I say I need payroll software installed at home.

December 5: We are at eleven weeks now. I take my first flights since the 9/11/01 terrorist attacks. High security at airports, with armed National Guard. These are also my first flights while pregnant and I do fine. At the NAMCA Christmas party at the Ritz Carlton in Marina del Rey, I have to use the restroom seven times! I decide to tell Claudia before the party starts, thinking she may be suspicious as to why I'm not drinking.

December 7: I tell Jesus this week, mainly because he guesses (says he could tell because of my tummy, but Leticia had told him not to say anything, because it wouldn't be polite).

December 14: At 12½ weeks now, I take Tracey and Tina to lunch to tell them my big news. They promise not to say anything around the office until I announce it. They are so excited for us. Tina tells me that Shanda had already guessed. After the goodbye happy hour for Janell, apparently Shanda said she thought I was "hiding something". Very perceptive woman!

December 15: I definitely have a growing tummy now. Elastic pants only, in size 16. I'm feeling disappointed in my pre-pregnancy weight (183.5). I had originally wanted to start my pregnancy at 15 pounds lower (165-170 range). Tonight is our first time babysitting for Jason and Alisa so they can attend his work Christmas party. This is great experience for us and I'm so glad to have the opportunity to spend time with the girls. As Scott sits with Lauren, I'm proud to be able to get Kayden to stop crying by rocking and soothing her.

December 16: I tell Bruce at SunSounds and e-mail Tracy.

December 17: I tell Ronee and e-mail Dan today…. At 11:30 p.m. I have pinkish red bleeding. VERY SCARY.

December 18: Thirteen weeks. More light bleeding at 7:15 a.m., still pinkish red. Call Dr. McN.'s answering service at 7:50 a.m. When I speak to the nurse, she says no big worry until bleeding gets very heavy (i.e. fills a pad in 15 minutes) or I have cramps. She is very blasé about it while I feel scared. She hears this all the time, but I'm a wreck. Brownish discharge all day, like the last day of my period. We mail out-of-state Christmas cards, trying to time it so they arrive right at Christmas with our news.

December 19: Very light brownish discharge continues.

December 20: Discharge almost gone. Scott's Christmas party. We tell Joe and Ali.

December 21: I announce our news to the rest of my coworkers, following our Christmas party at Macayo's Ahwatukee. Fun! Light brown discharge continues for another week.

December 24: Most folks have now received our Christmas card and letter. We sent out 61 of 'em and included our news!

December 25: Fourteen weeks and end of our first trimester. Unfortunately, I've gained more weight than I would have hoped, likely attributable to all the holiday treats and chocolates around the office. I've gained ten pounds already.

January 3, 2002: Fifteen weeks now. This is so exciting! At 12:20 p.m. we have our 2nd OB appointment. I love how Scott wants to go with me to my checkups. Today we hear this baby's heartbeat for the first time! Dr. McN. says my cervix looks fine and everything is good! Scott: "Wow!! Bah bom bah bom—It sounded so cool. I feel better after talking to the doctor."

January 9: Sixteen weeks and nearly sixteen pounds up. OK, I'm back from the buffets in Vegas. And the scales show a big jump: I'm at 199 now, one snack away from the 200 mark. Suck it up. You're pregnant and can't do a thing about it. Be thankful for no dreaded morning sickness.

January 13: Today I spend most of the day volunteering at my two side jobs, in which I continue to remain active. I also squeeze in a trip to Babies 'R Us and open our registry with just a couple items. By the evening, I'm exhausted.

January 16: 17 weeks now. Scott is referring to me as his "pod". We go to the Phoenix Suns game and now I find it very tiring to go up all those flights of steps to the upper deck. I'm feeling so out of shape! I'm tired in the evenings, like in my first trimester.

January 25: 18 weeks and 3 days. Today is our ultrasound at Tempe Imaging. I'm required to drink 44 oz of water between 1:45-2:15 and hold it until 3:30 (1st potty break), 3:45 (2nd potty break) and 4:15 (final potty break). Holding this much water brings me to tears; it's so uncomfortable that it's painful. But we get to see the baby for the first time since ten weeks! (Personally I thought the vaginal ultrasound had a clearer picture) Our due date of 6/25/02 is confirmed. We get to see: hands, feet, face, arms, legs, spine and, briefly, the heart beating! The technician says she's 80% sure it could be a boy! So, a little Angus, Jake, Anthony, still contemplating names…. Scott: "It was so cool to see the little legs kick and the arms move. It is just beyond words. Wow!!"

January 29: Nineteen weeks. Doctor's appointment today. I am diagnosed with marginal placenta previa. It's a partial block of the cervix by the placenta. The placenta probably will move, but if not we will need to have a c-section. Under doctor's orders, no intercourse until our next ultrasound because of this situation (six weeks from now).

February 2: So tired this evening because of such a busy Saturday. In preparation for our Super Bowl party, I spend 2½ hours cooking and cleaning. Then I make a trip to the gym, where they are kind enough to point out that it's my first appearance in 53 days. We have guests from 3-9 p.m. Fun but tiring!

February 5: 20 weeks, 23 lbs up. Half way! I'm not sure but maybe I felt a "twitch" yesterday—or if I just had it in my head because someone asks me everyday: "Have you felt the baby move yet?"

Grandma's thoughts of 2/5/02...

I've been thinking about boys lately (just in case). I've been observing the boys in my class & trying to tune into them in a different way (like a grandma—my secret—they don't know I'm doing this). I've discovered these things: they're very sweet and sensitive—maybe even need more strokes than girls—need reassurance about their future and their talents and who they are—they're very competitive with each other—at this age they're even more innocent than girls—they are often perfectionists—they love games & competition—they're loyal—they need a lot of security and parenting. They need to know & express love, sensitivity, and deep feelings just as much as girls do. You're probably saying, "You've taught for 31 years and you're just discovering boys????" Yes, I always knew they were here—but now I'm thinking to myself, "What do boys really need? What are their characteristics? How can I be the best possible grandma if that precious being is indeed a boy?" (I feel automatically comfortable about girls.)

February 7: Credit meeting in Long Beach. While waiting for Caroline to pick me up afterwards, I do some shopping and purchase two important items: baby book and "going home from the hospital" outfit. It's adorable and I don't care that it cost $25 because that's what my baby will first wear, other than hospital clothes. I learned in one of my books that it's best to have a pants outfit for going home in, not a gown, because of the car seat straps. I am feeling more very small "twitches" and because of the sheer number of them, I do think it is the baby moving.

February 17: 21½ weeks now. Bad spring allergies all week. Hard because most medications are to be avoided during pregnancy. Everything comes down to weighing the possible risk to the baby and my own health and comfort....

February 24: Visit Bandelier National Monument in New Mexico with Mom and Heidi, on the way back to Albuquerque after our "last" visit to Alamosa. Me trying to read the visitor's guide aloud while walking up the steps is pretty funny. I'm so short of breath now. It's sure nice to be home in my own cozy bed with my nice husband!

February 26: 23 weeks now. This morning I wake up with a bloody nose and am also spitting up blood. It's hard to swallow. Allergies?...Yesterday was five years since our very first date at Red Robin. Scott had softball last night, so tonight we go to Red Robin in Scottsdale for a commemorative dinner and, to make the evening extra special, Neal is our waiter!

February 27: Dr. McC. said "no" on taking Claritin, but Dr. McN. says okay. Sounds like a medical judgment call. I need allergy relief! Also have an Rx for a suppository, for a bacterial infection. Our ultrasound is scheduled for March 13 before we leave for our spring break San Diego trip.

March 2: After taking Claritin for two days, I switch to Sudafed, which is "safe" during pregnancy. I really can't tell if either one is effective enough to bother taking the medication risk.

March 5: Michael Owen is born in Virginia. He just has a few months' head start on Jake. Maybe they can play someday! We're at 24 weeks now. And I've now got the congestion yuck and sinus headache. Wonder if it's still just allergies?

March 9: Mackenzie's 8th birthday. Heidi and Bill leave for London and Switzerland. I'm not too miserable with allergies and congestion now...just moderately.

March 12: 25 weeks. I have heartburn most days now. I've never really had this before so it's all new to me!

March 13: Today is our 2nd lab ultrasound at 8:45 a.m. The tech says she's 99.9% sure he is a boy! There was a good "view" today. Also, good news: they confirmed the placenta has moved higher.

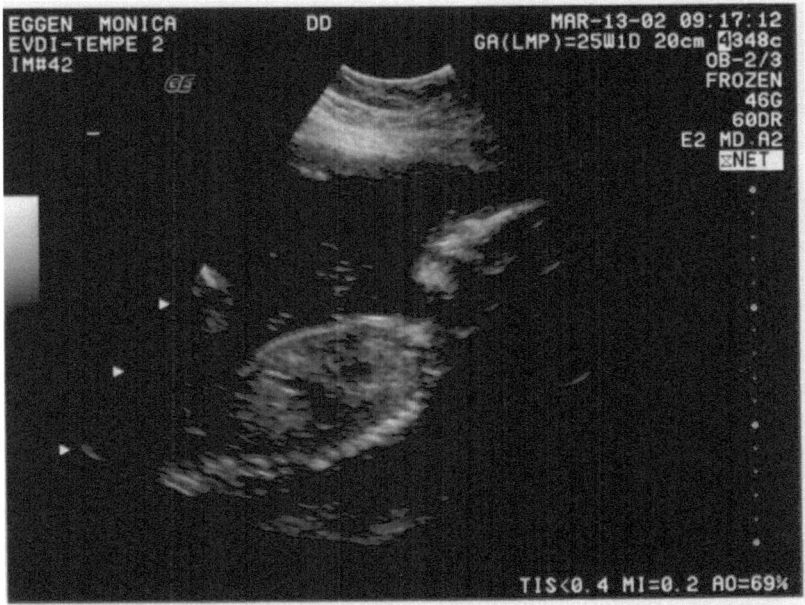

March 19: Now we are at 26 weeks and I've got the first noticeable swelling in my ankles.

March 22: I'm sick today and throw up at 9 a.m., for the first time during my pregnancy. I manage to go in to work for just one hour, but at least I tried. Unfortunately, I suffer from upset tummy most of the day, with a fever of 99.9°. I take Tylenol and Kaopectate at 9 p.m. These are on my doctor's list of "safe" medications. I'm disappointed that I can't go to our department's annual spring training game to see the Angels.

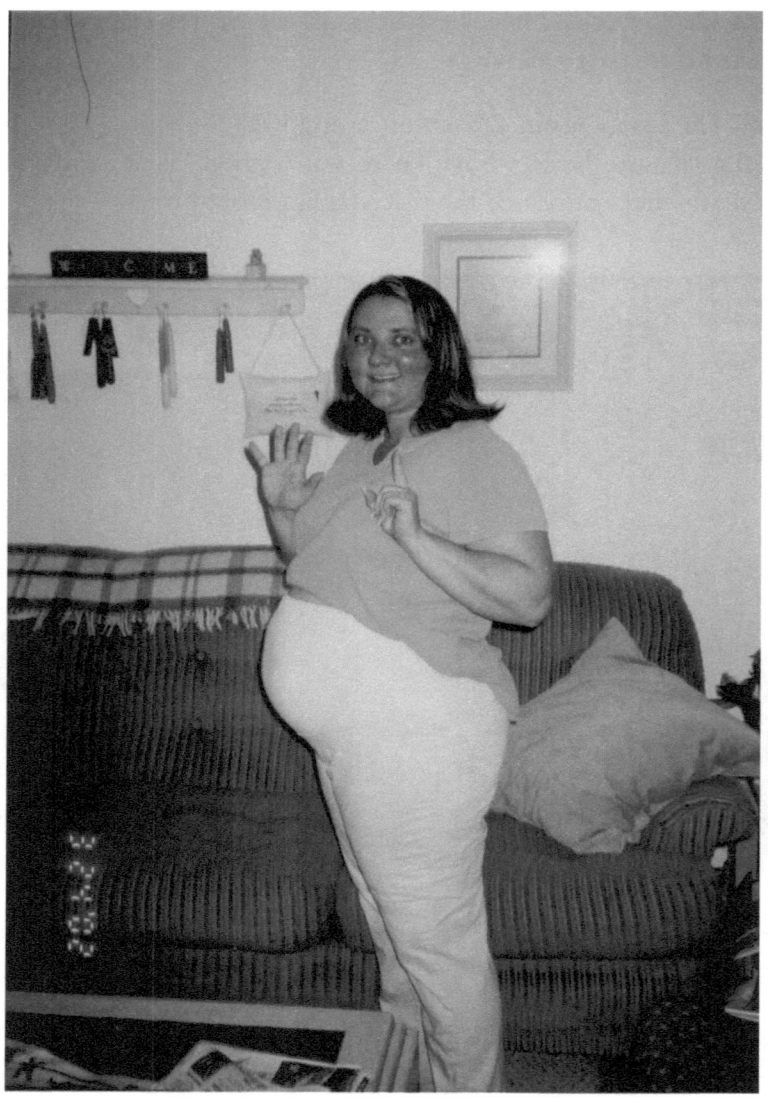

March 25: One day short of 27 weeks, Scott finally feels the first "external" baby kick, at the Olive Garden! Big day!!!

March 26: Today is the first doctor's appointment Scott has had to miss, due to taking a continued education class this month. Dr. McN. says sugar looks okay and no anemia. We start doctor's appointments at two week intervals now!...We see Crosby Stills Nash & Young at America West Arena this evening. Great show! I try to avoid the secondhand marijuana smoke (ha).

March 27: My last flight during this pregnancy.... Tracey and I fly to LA to visit CDM. We spend a lovely afternoon at Manhattan Beach.

April 2: Diamondbacks Ring Ceremony before the game tonight.... Mary and I go, and of course this baby 28 weeks *in utero*. As the team doctor, Dr. McC. gets a World Series ring, too. I can't wait to see it in person!

April 6: Baby Shower for Jake! (is that his name for sure?) It's an awesome party, at Heidi and Bill's clubhouse, and we have 35 people!

April 9: 29 weeks now, just 11 to go! Our doctor's appointment today begins the two-week visits. I have a sharp pain in my tummy at 8:45 a.m. Very scary! Dr. McN. diagnoses it as a ligament stretching between the two vertical abdominal muscles. Tomorrow I'm "32½" years old!

April 20: Today Scott and I attend our first Childbirth Preparation Class, near Mesa Lutheran Hospital. And this evening we assemble our new crib. It's beautiful butternut wood. Note to self: always assemble a large piece of furniture in the room it's meant to be in, so you don't have to disassemble it to get it through the door...one of many life lessons we'll be learning as we go.

April 22: We mail 38 thank-you cards for our shower gifts.

April 23: 31 weeks along now. New development: numbness in right middle finger. I learn that it may be carpal tunnel related to pregnancy and that it will likely go away after delivery.

April 27: 7 months now! Today Scott, Sean and I finish the assembly of our changing table. This was a challenging project, but when you follow directions it isn't difficult. Now our nursery furniture is all ready! I'm so excited. We really like this changing table. Also today I wash all the baby clothes, blankets and washcloths. The clothes fit in my old dresser perfectly. This is a good thing, because since we have decided to keep the guest bed in the nursery, there is no room for a larger dresser. Big deal today: I buy size 8 shoes for the first time in my life. I just had to get some shoes because mine don't fit anymore! The baby and I go to Scott's city track meet at MCC today. It's neat being pregnant and being there with him, seeing his students and their families.

April 28: Today, Scott packs our picnic basket and takes me for a wonderful picnic at the Tempe Town Lake, which I got to request from my "I Love You Coupons". Scott gave me these for the "paper" theme on our 1st anniversary.

May 2: At 32 weeks, all attempts to get my wedding ring off have now failed. It's really lodged on my finger now, indenting it. I do regret not taking it off back in cold Colorado in February. Now, do we resort to cutting it off…?

May 3: Today I have an appointment with Dr. McC. to get a wrist brace to try to alleviate my carpal tunnel symptoms. My numbness has gotten progressively worse and now my fingers are often tingly.

May 4: We attend our third childbirth preparation class today and get a chance to tour Mesa Lutheran Hospital! This is great because now we have a much better idea of what to expect and we can visualize exactly where we'll be. We had the opportunity to walk along the maternity ward, go in a labor/delivery/postpartum room, and peek into the nursery.

May 5: This is a busy weekend. Today I visit Target, do my recording at SunSounds and then trek all the way to Waddell to see my foster kids. I'm gone from 9:30 a.m. to 6 p.m. Very long day.

May 7: I'm now 33 weeks and up more than 45 lbs. I'm going to probably have my ring cut off. There's no hope for getting it off. Yesterday and today are the most swollen my feet and ankles have been. My feet are very swollen but I don't seem to have any other signs of toxemia. My blood pressure is 134/78 and I have no protein in my urine. I'm very thankful. My feet are so puffy that I have no shoes that fit, but soaking in the pool and sleeping with my feet up on a pillow does seem to help.

May 21: We are 35 weeks now—so close!!! I now begin weekly doctor's visits. Today is the 2nd most swollen day, next to May 7th. I have only missed two days in the pool since 5/7 and thanks to that and elevating my feet at night, the swelling is under control. Our pool is 80-82° and most refreshing! At our doctor's appointment today, Dr. McN. tests for Beta strep, which is dangerous to the baby. We'll have the results next week. She also sends us to the hospital for a "non-stress-test" as a precaution, to be sure the baby's movement is good. It is. She had asked if I feel him ten times between getting up and dinner. I'm not sure. ☺ It's so hard to be aware of movement while I'm at work. Plus it helps to lie down, like I was doing at the hospital, and he tends to kick more in the evenings, anyway. He is a late "sleeper-inner" in the mornings! I still have numbness in my fingers on my right hand. I'm not really sure if the wrist brace (that I'm supposed to wear at night and whenever possible during the day) does a darn thing!

May 28: 36 weeks, which is considered full-term! Yesterday was Memorial Day and it's in the 90°s. Today I see the nurse practitioner instead of Dr. McN., who is out sick. This cervix check is very uncomfortable, because I think she does it a bit differently. I even have some spotting afterwards. She reports that I am less than 1 cm dilated. It turns out that I do have Group B strep so they'll give me antibiotics in an IV before delivery to keep it from transmitting to the baby. I don't return to work after seeing the doctor at noon. I take a ½ sick day because I'm tired and have swollen feet.

May 29: Today I have pretty bad swelling in both my hands and feet. I have to wear slippers to work. Now both my hands are numb and tingly.

May 30: Still having swelling in the morning, which is considered a little more dangerous than evening swelling, because the feet have been elevated all night and this should have reduced any swelling. It appears there is very little I can do to fight it now. I'm still elevating my feet and soaking in the pool.

June 4: This is the month we've been waiting for! We are so excited! Well, swollen feet are just the rule now. In fact, slippers are my usual footwear! My 37-week doctor's appointment is cancelled due to Dr. McN. being called in to perform an emergency surgery.

June 6: We are watching a movie tonight when I start having sharp pains around 11 p.m., near or behind my pubic bone.

June 8: I'm having the pains again. I call Dr. McN., using the after-hours answering service since it's Saturday. She explains that there is some cartilage which slightly separates as we near delivery.

June 11: 38 weeks and the anticipation is growing! I am 60% effaced and still slightly less than 1 cm dilated.

June 15, 2002: This morning Scott and I are awakened by the ringing phone at 7:30 a.m. It's Sean. What's he doing calling so early? All of a sudden I feel a lot of wetness and I announce this to Scott, who quickly ends the call. My water has broken! When I get up, I continue to leak slightly. The time has come! Scott is not 100% convinced that the fluid is amniotic, but I convince him that we need to prepare to go to the hospital. This is ten days early! We learned in our class that once the water breaks, the baby must be delivered within 24 hours because his "balloon" is no longer intact and there is risk of infection. I don't feel any contractions. We take our time cleaning the waterbed, packing, showering, eating breakfast. We know there is really no rush. One more weighing-in shows I topped out at a 61.5-lb weight gain during this pregnancy. (Next time maybe I can be more careful during my first trimester!) We arrive at the hospital at 9:30 a.m. I am 1 cm dilated and 80% effaced. The nurse starts the Pitocin to induce labor at 10:30 a.m. In early afternoon, my contractions begin getting painful and very effective. I request an epidural. While we are waiting for the anesthesiologist, the nurse offers me a half-dose of painkiller. I don't refuse, although this isn't what the birth plan is. I don't want the baby to be drowsy from my painkiller and be unable to nurse. The dilating is moving quickly. When Scott returns from making a report to our many visitors about my progress, he is told that I've already dilated further! Around 5 p.m. we are shocked to find out that it's already time to start pushing. Due to the epidural, I feel nothing and am just "going through the motions"! I push when the nurse tells me I'm having a contraction—I wouldn't otherwise know! The delivery goes very smoothly. Jake is born at 6:07 p.m.!!!!!!!! Scott cuts the cord. What an incredible little baby! He's perfect and beautiful. I'm feeling slightly drugged and funky, not only from the experience of childbirth and knowing that he who was in me is now out of me, but also due to the lingering effects of the painkiller. After our first few minutes alone as a family, we invite our guests to join us. We have thirteen friends and family members waiting in the visitors' area who are very eager to see little Jake. The nursing staff is very patient with us. After an hour or so of ogling and Jake getting his first bath in the nursery, we are transferred to another LDRP room. At this point I need food, since I have had nothing since breakfast. About 9 p.m. Sean, our faithful "runner", brings back yummy Nello's pizza for a well-deserving mom and coach. The nursing staff helps us with the baby, although he will "room in" with me. The only place for Scott to rest in the room is a not-very-cozy recliner. We decide that it's best if Scott sleeps at home tonight because it's only a mile away and he may as well get a good night's sleep. Then he can spend lots of time with Jake tomorrow and help take care of him. I'm really not sure how much I'll be able to sleep with a newborn "five hours into the world", plus nurses coming in regularly to check on us. We say goodbye to Daddy…Jake and Monica are on their own for a few hours! No luck getting a good latch-on tonight. It's scary for me—when will Jake get something to eat after such a long day? We get comfortable and settle in for the night.

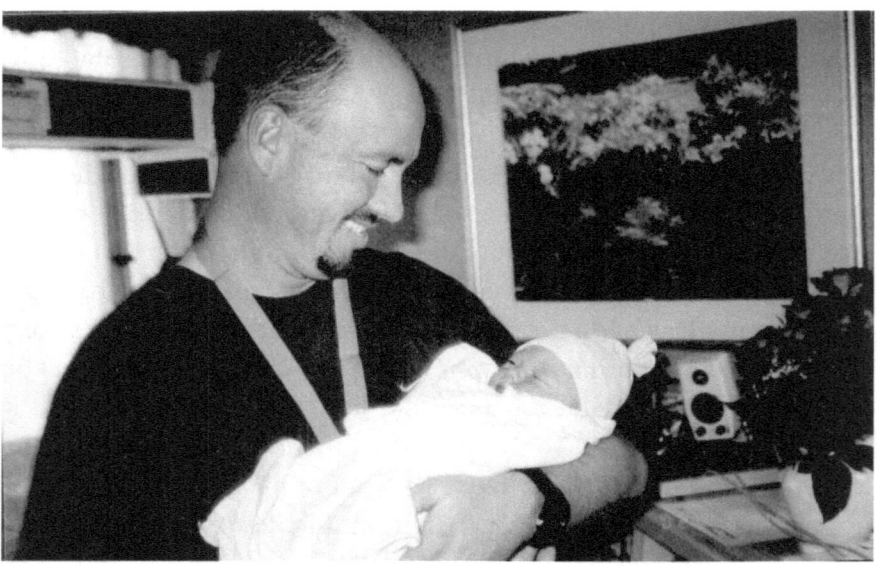

Part II:
After Jake Arrives

June 16, 2002: Sometime after midnight, the nurse checks to see if Jake has been able to latch-on and eat yet. "Not yet," is my reply. She explains that she'll check his blood sugar and if it's too low, they'll need to feed him some supplementary formula. This is the case. He gets to eat 1 oz of formula. At his 5:30 a.m. feeding, Jake latches on successfully!!! Yeah!!!! We did it! *From now on, all he eats is breastmilk until he is six months old!* I am so grateful for the nursing staff at Mesa Lutheran Hospital, giving me support and latch-on tips to help with this challenging first 12 hours. Today is Sunday and we will have a "parade of visitors" before the day is out. It's wonderful and there are so many people who are happy and excited about Jake's arrival.

June 17: On this second night in the hospital, when the nurse takes Jake to the nursery for his hearing tests in the middle of the night, I don't argue when she offers to keep him for a few hours so I can get some sleep. However, my sleep is fitful and although I know that we are the only ones who have a matching security band and can take him out of the hospital, I still have anxiety and nightmares that he has been taken. This mother/child bond is unexplainable. When he is all wrapped up in his blanket and his little head is all that is peeking out, he reminds me of a butter bean and this will be his nickname for months to come. This is our "going home" day! Moms and babies now stay in the hospital for 48 hours following the birth. That means we should be checking out by around 6 p.m. today. Dr. McN., who still hasn't seen the baby because she was unavailable for the delivery, is running late and doesn't make it to check on us until after 6 p.m. We start packing and I nibble on some dinner. It takes a long time. Scott has a softball game tonight and he really wants to go. I feel a little stressed about him getting there on time. I need to be sure that we are okay with Baloo before he leaves. We don't know how he's going to react and I don't know where to be safe in the house. Jake is just so tiny—less than 7 lbs—and Baloo is 100 lbs! He can crush him with his paw without realizing it. We may need to keep him outside, but it's just so hot for such a big, furry dog. With the packing, the planning and the uncertainty of how to get all our stuff to the car plus use the carseat for the first time, the nurse decides she needs to monitor my blood pressure a little longer, since it's a little high now. We finally leave around 8 p.m. Jake is such a little guy in a big carseat! He's adorable in his special white two-piece going home outfit (that will never fit him again). The nursing staff wheels Jake and me to the curb in a wheelchair. Scott has so many gifts and flowers to take to the car, plus all my stuff. Finally we make the mile drive home and show Jake around his house, introducing Baloo and Jake at 8:30 p.m. Baloo is very curious, but Scott is very careful. He gets us all oriented and set up, then takes his leave to go late to softball.

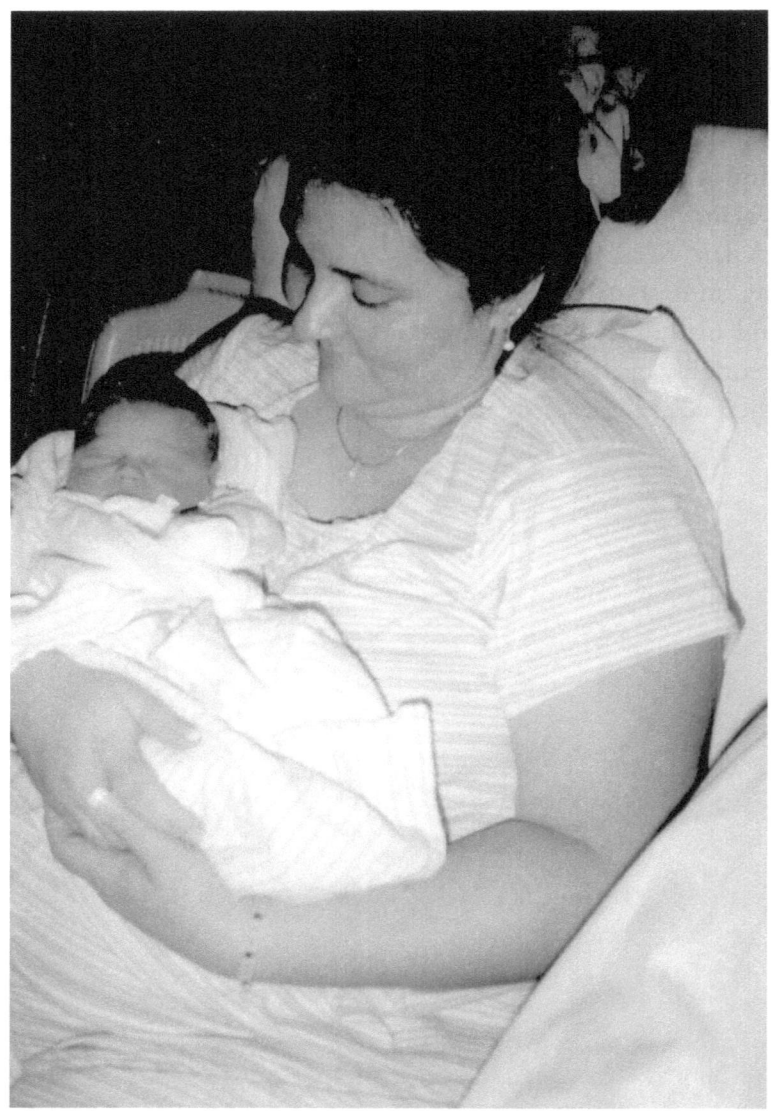

June 18: Today I have my first hint of milk. I've been feeding Jake colostrum since his first latch-on.

June 19: Today I "GOT MILK"! My breasts are engorged so it's pretty obvious. Today is Jake's first doctor's appointment. He weighs 6-2. They send us to the lab to check his bilirubin levels, which are at 19. Dr. A., filling in for Dr. C-M., prescribes phototherapy for Jake's mild jaundice. The sunlamp "suitcase" arrives at 9 p.m. and we're supposed to leave him in it "24-7" unless he's eating or we are changing his diaper. He also has a sunbelt that he can wear when we are holding him. He's so tiny in that suitcase, but seems fairly comfortable. The lights are warm so it probably feels good. Scott is sleeping in the living room with Jake, under the glow of the sunlamp.

June 20: Jake has to go back to the lab again today for another blood test. His bilirubin levels are improving and are at 13. Today he actually sleeps through the blood test because of a very gentle lab technician. Tonight will be his second night on lights. Today I make a 1 oz bottle for Scott to feed Jake! And a second one for nighttime, so I don't have to get up. Jake has no problem taking the bottle and is doing fine still eating from me.

June 21: Today is Jake's third bilirubin test and we make good use of our new pacifier. He is allowed to get off the lights and they come to pick them up at 9 p.m. Today I make Scott his third bottle because I'll be out at Nello's and BestFed with Heidi from 10 a.m.-2 p.m. I miss Jake and it's hard to be gone that long, but good for me to have a break. Today I'm having serious engorgement. I try warm compresses and some manual expression, in order to be more comfortable. Heidi says I need to buy the pump now and not worry about trying them out. She gets it for me.

June 22: Jake is one week old! We have our (usual) "parade of visitors" which today includes Grandpa Larry, Grandma Carol, Beth, Pat and Taylor, Marilyn, Grandma Elaine and John ("Gramps"). In between all that visiting, Jake has his very first sponge bath!

June 23: My swelling has finally decreased in my feet. And just for fun I weigh: 10 lbs less than last Saturday (that seems rather anti-climactic since Jake was 7 of it). Jake's first social outing tonight: he comes with us to our co-ed softball game at Tempe Diablo Park!

June 24: Scott now calls Jake a "boobsucker". I start a breastfeeding log because it's too hard to keep track of his feedings. I simply cannot remember when he last ate. This works out really well and I continue it for months. It also helps Scott to know when his last feeding was and how much he ate.

June 25: More often than not, we host the "parade of visitors" daily! Today's starts with Uncle Duane and Mackenzie, then Grandma and Gramps, then Jesus and Leticia and finally Grandpa and Uncle Sean.

June 26: Jake's umbilical cord falls off!

June 27: Today is Jake's second doctor's appointment. He now weighs 7-4. His next well-baby appointment will be at two months. Today we visit Grandma's for the first time.

June 28: Jake slept 4½ hours last night!!! ☺ My fingers are still numb, but the good news is that my bleeding is finally reducing. Scott and I venture out for dinner to the Blue Adobe, with Jake in his carseat. Jake sleeps the entire time!

June 29: Today we mail Jake's birth announcements. We attend the wedding of Joe and Ali. Grandma babysits for five hours. Jake has his 4th and 5th bottles ever.

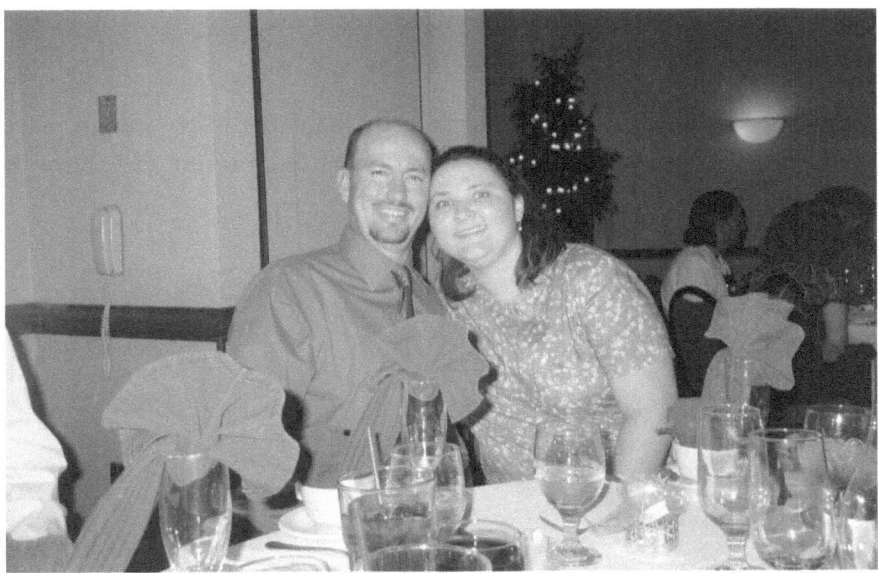

June 30: Big day: Jake's first Eggen Sunday dinner at Mary's! Also, he joins us at co-ed softball again in the evening in over 100° heat. Even though he wears a cool outfit and I keep him sprayed with cool water, the heat makes me nervous.

July 1: My bleeding is seriously tapering off now. Yeah! Tonight Jake attends his first Arizona Diamondbacks game. The Dodgers beat the D'backs. Jake sleeps most of the game in the BabyBjörn. For the very first time, I nurse him in a public area. We have seats in the Infiniti level for a few games and this level has a nice elevator lobby that I am directed to…. It's relatively private and I manage to survive.

July 2: Scott now refers to me as "The Chow Wagon", which is a rather unique term of endearment. Mary babysits today so Scott and I can escape to a matinee. We see *Minority Report*.

July 3: It's nice to have my feet back to their normal condition. Today I resume our weekly family walk with Dad and Heidi. We've been "walking" Dad now for several years. And now Jake joins us in the Björn for his very first walk at Fiesta Mall.

July 4: Today Jake has his first bath in the baby bathtub! We can place it on the kitchen counter and we have just enough room. He seems to enjoy it!

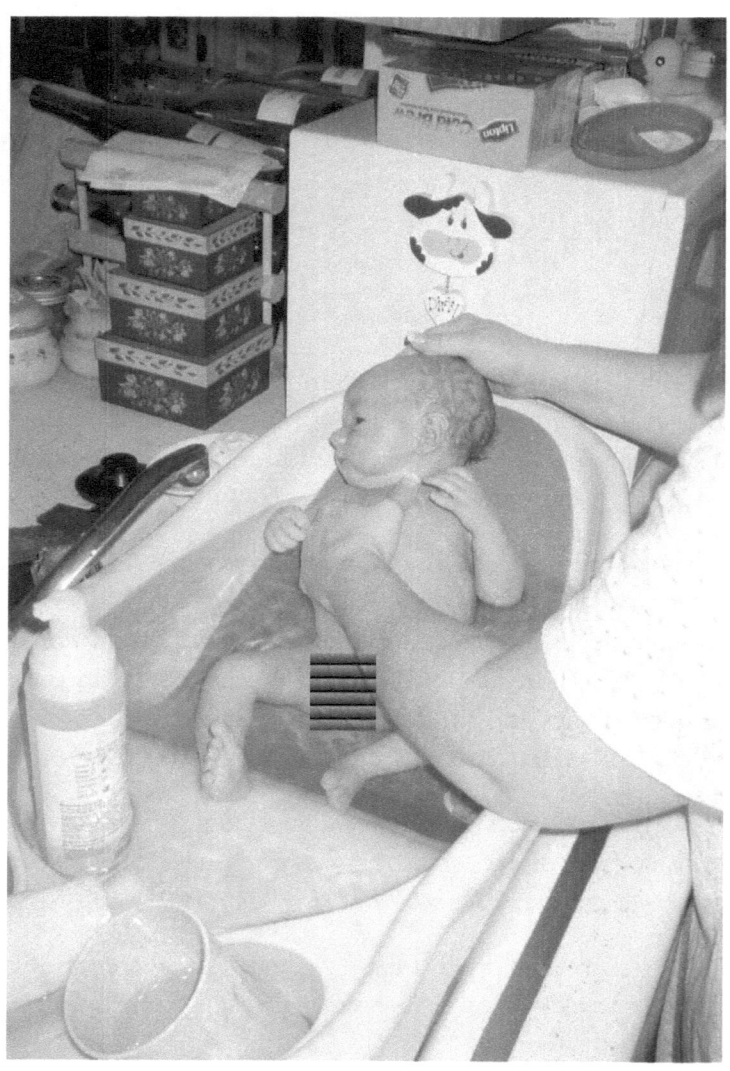

July 5: I go out to lunch with Heidi today. This is lunch #3 since Jake. We've been having lunch once a week for nearly four years! Jake cries a lot today—the worst crying spell so far. My bleeding still continues to taper off gradually.

July 6: Jake is three weeks old today! And today is my first trip to the gym! I walk 30 minutes on the treadmill, happy as a clam with my *Girlfriend's Guide to Surviving the First Year of Motherhood*.

July 8: By six a.m. this morning, I've spent exactly half an hour in bed during the night. Jake generally wakes up hungry and wants to nurse twice during the night. We nurse in the rocker/recliner and as I'm rocking him back to sleep, I fall asleep! This is why I'm not getting much sleep in bed, horizontally, these days. Since we have a waterbed, he can't sleep with us, otherwise we could nurse and fall back to sleep there. Today I buy a third nursing bra (42E) and a sports bra in my current size (40DD). Those sizes sound frightening! I do a lot of Omni-iMount work today, including payroll data entry.

July 9: Better night last night: we slept in the nursery and I made a special effort not to fall asleep in the living room. I'm still bleeding but it's very light now. Today Jake has his second bath! It's fun and he really seems to enjoy it. I've decided I can't use the bath gloves I bought (for washing slippery babies), because I must touch his soft skin!

July 11: Today is Jake's 2nd walk at the mall: Scottsdale Fashion Square this time, in the Björn, with Grandpa and me.

July 12: Today Scott and I make Jake's hand casting mold. It's really cool. Jake weighs 10 lbs today on our digital scale (rounded to tenths). We may go to the baby scale at BestFed. Tonight Scott is going to relieve me of my feeding duties and the goal is for me to get to sleep all night for the first time in four weeks! I've pumped two bottles for him: 4 oz and 3 oz.

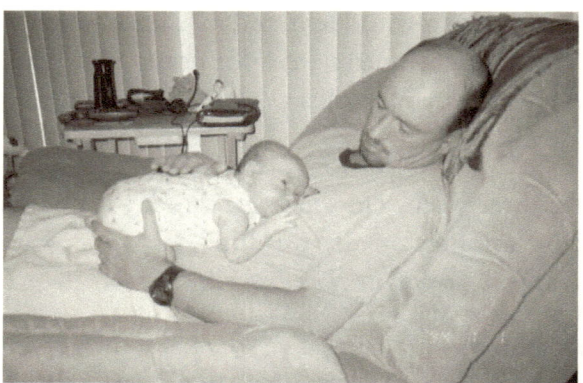

July 13: Our plan works! I get to sleep from 11 p.m. to 6 a.m.!!! And I didn't even move the whole night. I needed that desperately. Thanks, Scott!! Jake is four weeks old and my bleeding has finally, essentially stopped.

July 14: Today we visit Jason, Alisa and the girls so we can see their new playhouse. Jason is going to NASA for six weeks at the end of July! Alisa has offered to watch Jake from October until Christmas and then we'll re-evaluate. We have the Eggen Sunday dinner at our house tonight. Major monsoon afterwards. Heavy wind (or even a microburst) rips our roof off the east side of our house. Electrical fires across the street at Mesa Country Club. The power is out for over an hour. It's hot and muggy with no air conditioning, but I hate to open the doors because of the smoke outside. It's a strange summer night. I'm inside in a dark house with a tiny baby and it's scary. Finally we join Scott, Doug and Sean outside, even though it's smoky and the fire is just across the street.

July 15: At one month old, Jake weighs 10-7 at BestFed with clothes, so 10-4 without clothes.

July 18: Today we make our first trip to OmniMount since Jake was born! We spend an hour and 20 minutes visiting and letting my coworkers admire our cute baby. Tonight Jake and I watch Daddy play softball. This is Jake's very first time to an Eggen CPA game and he brings good luck. The team wins both tournament games.

July 20: Jake is five weeks old. He makes his first trip to Sky Harbor Airport, with Mom and Aunt Heidi. We pick up Aunties Stephanie and Caroline, who fly in from Chicago and Orange County, respectively. It's great to see them and introduce them to their first nephew!

July 21: Scott, Uncle Doug, Uncle Duane and Marc leave today for Torrey Pines. Last year I bought Scott a gift certificate for his birthday and he needs to use it before it expires. He didn't want to leave us for two days, but knows he'll have a good time with his family.

July 23: Today Jake goes to his 3rd mall: Chandler Fashion Center. Caroline has to go home today. Scott arrives home at 7 p.m. and we have another major monsoon. The roof leaks and water pours into our storage room, as we frantically funnel it out the door using a wheelbarrow to keep the room from flooding. Unbelievable.

July 24: Jake is sad today, or maybe has a bad tummyache. Scott assembles Jake's bouncy/vibrating seat—what a great idea!

July 25: Jake is now rounding to 11 lbs on our digital scale! He's sure growing fast! He's doing so well with breastmilk.

July 26: We discovered the "slow flow" nipple is much better for the bottle, otherwise Jake drinks too fast. Thanks for the idea, Grandma!

July 27: Today Jake is six weeks old and he stays at Grandma's for the first time: from 10 a.m. to 1:15 p.m., while Monica is at the hair salon and Scott is busy with the roofer who is putting on the "temporary roof". Jake entertains himself now in the bouncy seat! He loves music and lights. He's also very observant now and can "follow" objects several feet.

July 28: Jake makes his first trip to Tempe Town Lake today. Family walk in his stroller with Grandpa, Aunt Heidi and me.

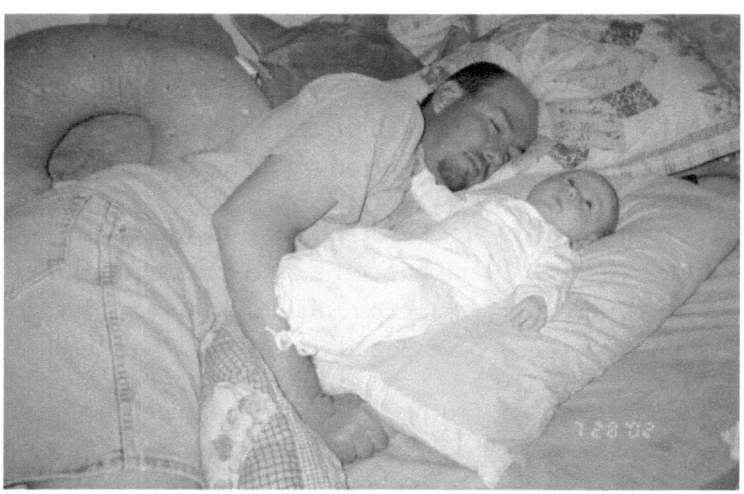

July 29: Just when I thought it was finally getting easier, why is breast-feeding hurting again? Today Jake has several periods of just sitting or laying and looking around…not crying, just looking around, absorbing, for up to ½ an hour each!

July 30: Jake now weighs in at 11½ lbs on our home scale. Scott and Jake accompany me to Surprise today to visit my CASA kids. We visited with them for an hour at their new foster-adopt home. This is Jake's longest excursion to date! (about 100 miles round trip)

July 31: Jake continues to be mesmerized by the light shining through the vertical blinds in the living room. We first noticed this several weeks ago.

August 1: This is our 2nd day "with swing". Jake sleeps in it for hours. I know it's not the most restful sleep, probably, but he sure likes it. Today, Jake, Scott and I have lunch at Chipotle and stroll around

Chandler Fashion Center. Fun! (even Scott thinks so and he's not a mall-lover!)

August 2: Last night, Jake slept for 4½ hours again. He's been getting better all this week with holding his head up! His neck muscles are very strong now. And he is absolutely adorable. Scott's summer vacation is quickly coming to a close. He and I escape to a movie again: *Signs*!

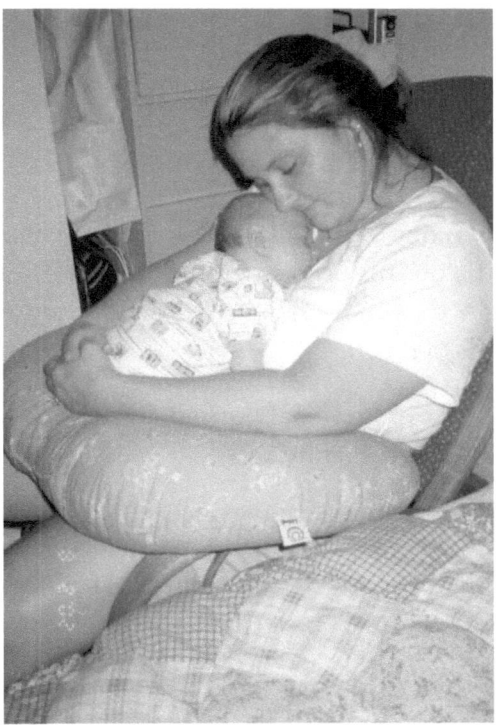

August 3: Jake is seven weeks old and it occurs to me we've never taken him to Grandpa and Grandma Pershall's house, although they've been over to visit at our house very regularly. Jake and I pay a visit there and then we go to Mall #4 together: Arizona Mills.

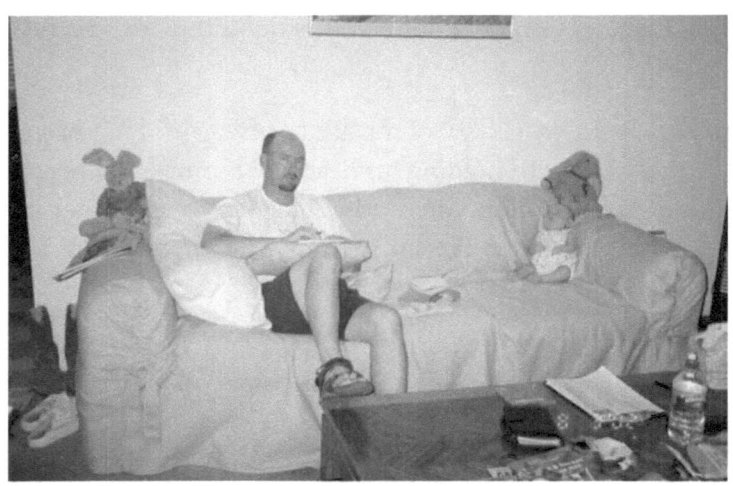

August 4: Today is our first family walk in our neighborhood with me, Scott, Jake and Baloo. It's been so hot; it just never sounds appealing. Scott and I begin to wonder if Jake will be a really verbal child. He grunts and "talks" so much!

August 5: Jake's first professional portrait, at Arizona Mills! Forever to be known as "The Angel Picture". ☺

August 6: Jake weighs 12½ lbs on our home scale!

August 7: Last night was my 3rd full night of sleep since Jake was born: 6½ hours! Scott gave Jake a bottle. Today I get Jake to smile!

August 8: When I am stuffing paychecks tonight, it occurs to me that my fingers aren't numb anymore!! Today Jake and I go to Babies 'R Us with Grandma. They have a nice Mom's room there for nursing.

August 9: Other than spending a few hours there, today is Scott's first day back at work. It was so wonderful that he was home with us for all of Jake's first eight weeks!!!! (other than the two days he was in San Diego) It was such a special time for us as a family and it made all the difference in the world, getting through this challenging (tiring) time as Team Eggen. We have a happy boy who smiled and giggled for Scott tonight in Prescott. This is Jake's first trip out of town!

August 10: We enjoyed our first night in our cottage. This morning we get up at 5 a.m. to drop Scott off at Antelope Hills Golf Course. Jake and I go to Coco's together for breakfast, then take a little nap. Later we walk down to the Arts Festival at the court house square before going out to the golf course to have lunch. Uncles Doug and Duane visit with us at our cottage and later in the evening we walk down to Whiskey Row with Jake in the stroller. He's fussy so we get take-out and eat back at the cottage.

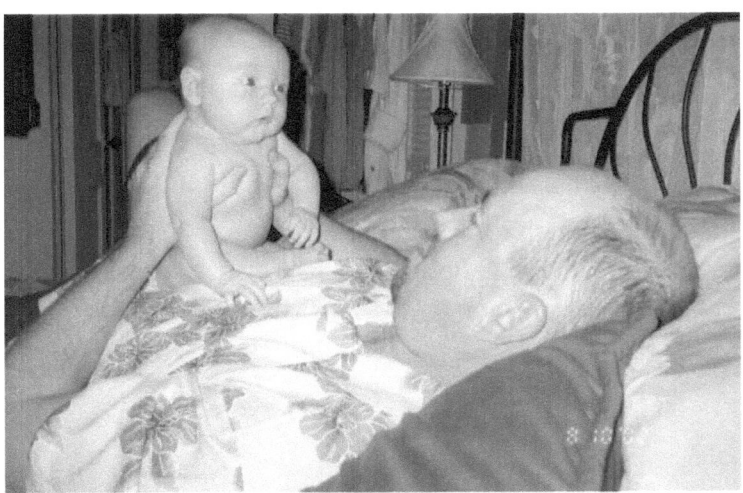

August 11: Last night we had a rough time getting a crying baby to stay asleep, but once he did, he actually slept 5½ hours!!!! This is a record! Jake also naps in the morning until 9 a.m. and sleeps all the way back to Phoenix. Uncle Bill and Aunt Heidi buy a new house!

August 12: I've officially lost half of my "baby weight"! (31 of 62 lbs gained during pregnancy) This has been accomplished with no real effort on my part: regular household activity, walking 1-2 times weekly and no special eating efforts. I have my postpartum doctor's appointment today and she says everything seems fine. She advises the "mini-pill" to be sure I don't get pregnant right away—no guarantees when you are breastfeeding. Could be from all the hormonal changes, but I've been diagnosed with bacterial vaginosis twice this year. As of today, I have just four weeks left at home with Jake before I go back into the office: the dreaded countdown begins.

August 13: Today is a very long day caring for Jake all by myself: on "baby duty" until 10:15 p.m. That's challenging, especially when you include errands out of the house. We go walking at Arizona Mills.

August 14: Jake's 2nd trip out of town! This time to Payson with Grandpa, Aunt Heidi and Mom. This is our first visit to Bill and Heidi's new condo because they closed the end of June, just after Jake's birthday.

August 15: Today we visit Woods Canyon Lake, where Grandpa and Aunt Heidi try to catch some fish. Jake sleeps in his stroller in the fresh mountain air for THREE hours! We arrive back home to Mesa at 7 p.m. Today Jake is two months old.

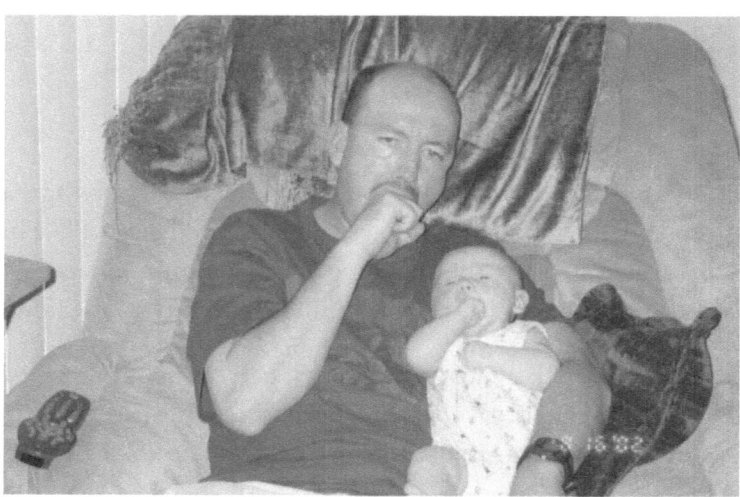

August 17: Nine weeks since Jake was born! He weighs 13-7 now, on the BestFed scale, and already wears 3-6 month clothes. He is sucking on his fist every day. It's very cute. Scott and I have declared Saturday "bottle night" until further notice, so I can get a full night's sleep at least once a week. Tonight we go out to dinner at BJ's at Chandler Mall with Kathy and Scott, who are expecting their first little one on October 13.

August 18: Jake slept 5 hours last night!!! I feel like I have a perpetual "to-do" list, but I do get some things done over the weekend. I'm really busy with OmniMount work right now. I've enjoyed *The Girlfriends' Guides* so much that I decide to e-mail Vicki Iovine to tell her how much they've helped me along! Jake has a rough evening, with a long crying spell. This is very rare, as he's not generally inconsolable. The "Daddy Dance" is the only thing that calms him down. Yeah, Daddy!!

August 19: I've made a commitment to myself to type up all these notes I've journaled…. Jake slept six hours last night! (to bed at 11:15 and I heard him crying at 5:25 a.m.) Now we wonder if this was a fluke or maybe due to the hour he spent crying last night? I wonder if that crying made him more tired.

August 20: Jake slept seven hours last night! (to bed at 11:15, then we all got up at 6:20 and he wasn't even crying) Now, was this a fluke? Was it the Tylenol? He didn't eat for eight hours.

August 21: Jake slept seven hours straight again last night! I hate to be skeptical that it's permanent but, truly, just last week he only went three hours. I'm absolutely swamped with OmniMount stuff this week, including payroll and processing new hires. This week my journal quotes George Ade from 1901: "Be it ever so humble, there's no place like home for wearing what you like"—and some days it's pajamas!

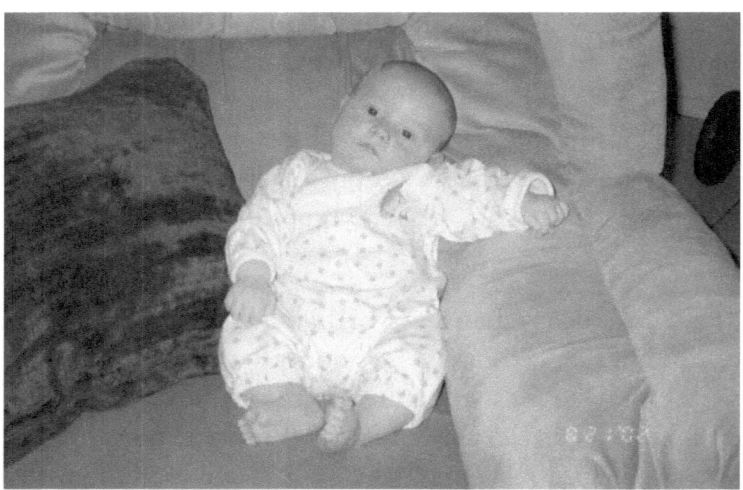

August 22: Today I sort boxes on the back patio. After our storage room flooded in the monsoon last month, Scott pulled everything out to dry and I only have a few boxes left to sort into save, toss, donate.

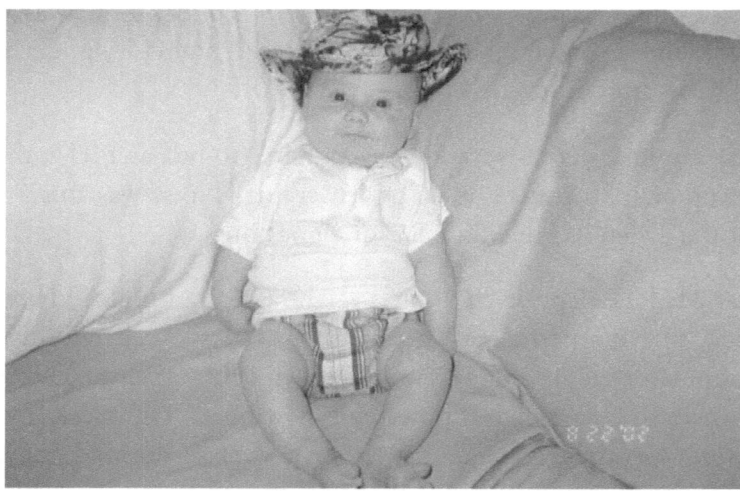

August 23: Today Jake's "Boobman" onesie arrives. I had to order it—too funny. Jake accompanies me to OmniMount (not wearing

that, of course), so I can drop off the payroll. Then we take a drive north and end up at Uncle Duane's office for a visit. Today is very unusual because Jake has two 50-minute nursing sessions. Also then he's up from 3 p.m. to midnight, with only one short nap. I'm having a little spotting from the mini-pill.

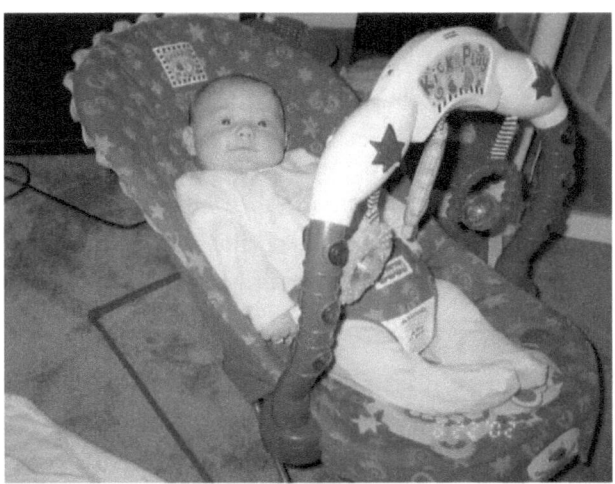

August 24: Today is Saturday and Jake is ten weeks old! I have a 40" waistline, but it continues to decrease with very little effort on my part, other than the big reason: breastfeeding. Tonight, after we return home from Joe and Ali's BBQ, we have Jake's first family swim session in our pool!

August 25: I have two weeks until I return to work. I'm working hard to mentally prepare myself. Today is Kathy's baby shower, which is really fun. Afterwards, I stop by the Mesa Main Library to pick up Jake's free book. We received a flyer for a "Storytime Lapsit" in September, 10 a.m. each Wed or Thurs. I was excited, but then sad because I can only take him the first week. I go back to work 9/9. Tonight is a big, scary night—I got up my guts and tried on my new sexy leopard print nightie!

August 26: Jake sometimes reaches out and touches us now. He had always done that when we nurse, though. He smiles more now, especially in the morning. Today just Jake and I take a morning walk with the Björn. It's getting to be a pleasant temperature in the mornings now (80°). Late night with Scott returning home from the first game of the fall softball season with Duane at 11 p.m.

August 27: For the last two nights, we've returned to 2 or 3 a.m. feedings but we are starting a plan to get Jake to bed by 11 p.m., back into his more "standard" schedule, which means last nursing at 10:30. I attend the OmniMount board meeting this afternoon, from noon—4 p.m. I think I'll try to come home for a lunchtime nurse when I first go back to the office. I had a very light period which ended today, which may be more spotting related to the mini-pill. I know I probably won't have a real one until I stop nursing.

August 28: Scott turns in his Request for FMLA today: to take during my first four weeks back to work (9/9-10/4). New roof going on today! The hammering is so loud, from 5:30 a.m. to 12:30 p.m. The afternoon peace and quiet is wonderful.

August 29: Roofing continues on the same schedule. We're so excited to have a brand new roof! I'm working really hard to make some headway on my "to-do" list. Today I type and format Jake's gift list for his baby book. It takes almost two hours. He's received so many gifts! I've also been trying to find time to send thank you cards, prepare and send wedding/birthday gifts, etc. Scott and I open a new CD with the proceeds from the sale of my house and start a college savings certificate for Jake with the interest from my previous CD. Scott and I close on our refinanced home equity loan (i.e., Scott's Jeep).

August 30: I love my baby boy! I **hate** to think about leaving him in just **10 days**! He is now 14 lbs, 2 oz.

September 1: I like this week's quote in my journal—by Randle Cotgrave in 1611: "Every bird likes its own nest best". It may be small and cluttered with baby things but it's cozy! Today, I finally finish repacking crates from the monsoon flood damage and completely clean the back patio. Yeah! Believe me, this is no small feat when either Scott or I need to be on "baby duty" 24-7, or arrange for a sitter, which we have had to do on occasion in order to fix the storage room up after the storm damage.

September 2: Today is Labor Day. Scott, Jake and I use this rare weekday off to run errands all morning, hitting Blockbuster, Home Depot, and the grocery store before dropping off yet another load of goodies at Savers for Big Brothers Big Sisters, our charity of choice. We spend the entire afternoon at Mary's for a family BBQ. I've started nursing in the guest bed at night instead of in the recliner, since I always end up falling asleep and spending the rest of the night in the recliner.

September 3: Today Jake and I go over the Arizona Mills to pick up the "Angel picture" and then go to Target. It's so hot. Grandpa, Heidi and Bill all visit later. Daddy thinks the "Angel picture" is a little silly, but I love it and intend to frame it!

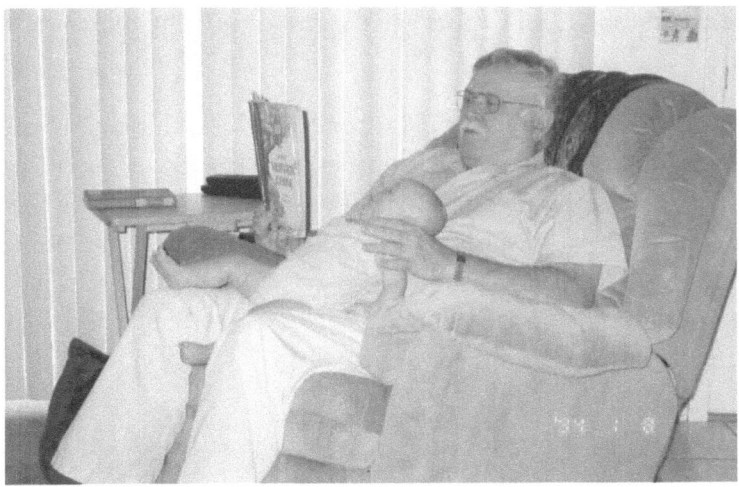

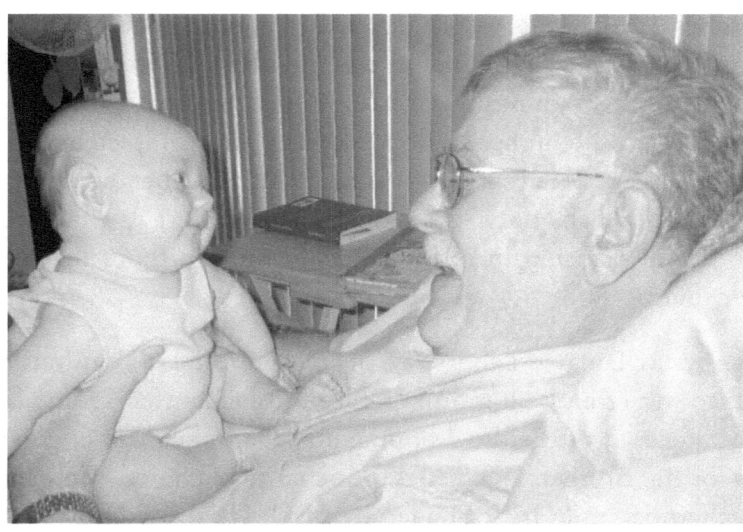

September 4: After I finish payroll this afternoon, I take Jake to the Family Resource Center's "First Steps Together" play group. There are about 8 parents there for infant play time. Lots of sanitized toys on quilts. It's fun! Later, from 4-6 p.m., I go over to OmniMount for a meeting on new projects and initiatives so I'm ready to jump in on Monday, my first day back to work full-time. I'm really focused on Jake right now, making the most of the "quantity" of time left. I love how sometimes Jake will "purr" at the end of nursing, when he's really contented and comforted.

September 5: Today Jake and I attend the Mesa Library's Storytime Lapsit for babies. We receive another free cardboard book just for going! That's a really nice program. It's so neat. Jake enjoys the songs and the other kids. Towards the end of the program, I'm close to tears because it hurts so much to go back to work and miss these times. Later in the afternoon, on a lazy, hot day, Jake, Aunt Heidi and I swim at Grandma's for the first time together.

September 6: Jake continues to sleep in his swing for long naps. His naps are usually 3 hours in the morning and 2-3 hours in the afternoon/evening. It's really nice!

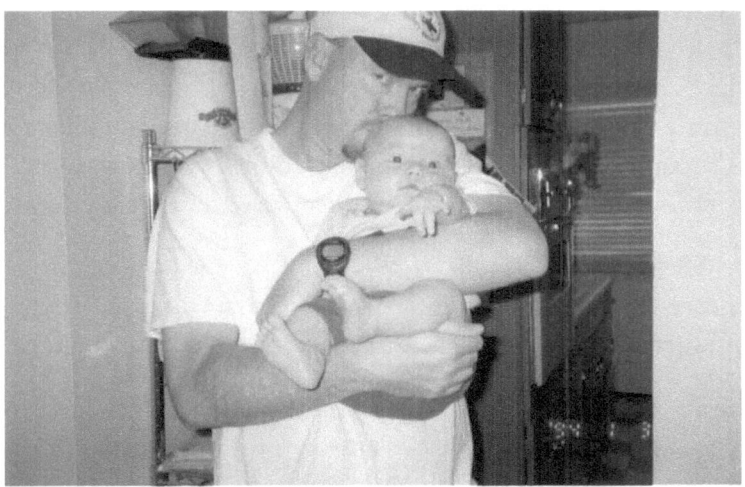

September 7: Jake is 12 weeks old today! He celebrates by throwing up for the first time, at 5:45 a.m. He also has a cough. Scott's actually had a cough for four weeks, but we didn't believe it was contagious. Now I have a sore throat, and I'm developing congestion and a runny nose. We sure hate to be sick around such a young baby. It's very rainy and "monsoony" today, and we drive all the way to Anthem for Taylor's birthday party. She's 3 now. The party gets moved inside because of the rain. On the way, we stop by Brad's new house in McDowell Mountain Ranch.

September 8: Today is Sunday and my last day at home with Jake before starting work full-time. I spend a really nice day at home with Jake and Scott. Our softball team, the Saki Bombers, is back in action starting tonight from 8-9 p.m. This is my first time playing since last summer, so that feels kind of strange. Finally, at 11 p.m., I'm on my way to bed. I expect to get up with Jake around 3 a.m., then my alarm will go off for work at 6:20 a.m. Thankfully, Scott's first day of FMLA begins tomorrow. This will be challenging, but not as much as if I had to pack Jake up and take him somewhere.

September 9: Jake surprises us by sleeping all night!!! This is the first time in weeks and I tell him "thank you". It's so nice to go back to work after actually getting a full night's sleep! Today at work I only concentrate on thoroughly cleaning my desk. Tracey and Claudia have done a super job of absorbing all the day-to-day workflow, so my inbox isn't overflowing, but I dust, clean, organize and get ready to get back into it.

September 10: Work is going much better than I anticipated. Seeing Jake at lunch is really helping. I'm pumping at work twice a day.

September 11: Today is the 1-year anniversary of 9/11. The country is saddened again. Last night Jake slept over 8 hours. In fact, I got up, pumped and showered before he stirred! So far I'm getting enough milk from pumping that I'm having a little extra to freeze and supplement my "stash".

September 12: Jake sleeps over 8 hours again! I only got 6½ because I have so many things to do, but I'm certainly not complaining! My pump batteries died today, so I need to do a better job of planning next week. I have rechargeable batteries because I was trying to avoid having to replace 8 batteries all the time. See, the only place for me to pump at work (the restroom) has no electrical outlet, so I'm stuck. Heidi and I see *Divine Secrets of the Ya-Ya Sisterhood*—my second time. What a great "escape" movie.

September 13: Today Scott is 35! I'm home on Fridays indefinitely: "on call" and checking e-mail. We have a doctor's visit for Jake today. He has a bit of a cold, with a cough and congestion. I honestly don't do a lick of work today besides checking my e-mail before we leave for the doctor's office. I make Scott dinner for his birthday, which he thinks is the only celebration. We get to freeze the excess milk from this workweek. This week was not awful, because I had a lot to do, including our big G/L project. The pumping routine isn't too bad.

September 14: John/Gramps suffers a very unfortunate injury today, breaking his leg near Ground Zero in NYC. We are desperately awaiting the latest news from Mom, who is on her own, dealing with the Manhattan hospital, St. Vincent's. Tonight I succeed in surprising Scott with 22 family and friends for a birthday party in the Pope Room of Buca di Beppo in Mesa. We have a fabulous time, although we certainly exceed the maximum capacity of the room.

September 15: Today Gramps has leg surgery, with pins inserted.... I end up pumping only twice all weekend. I know I need to nurse as often as possible when I am home with Jake.

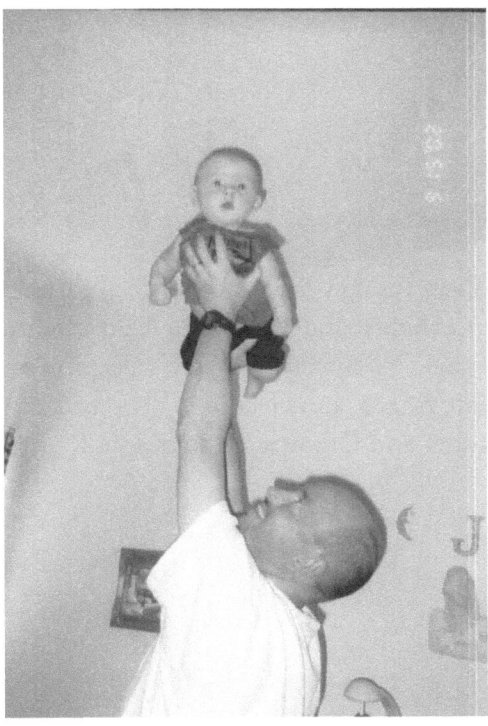

September 16: Today is Monday, and Scott starts his second week home alone with Jake. Jake is grabbing things now: our clothes and holding onto stuffed animals. It's so cute. Poor Grandma. She is living a nightmare. She is sleeping in Newark and commuting back and forth to Manhattan. Her car was broken into, while she was at the hospital.

September 17: We, along with Heidi and Bill, send flowers to Gramps' room today. Jake's cough sounds terrible.

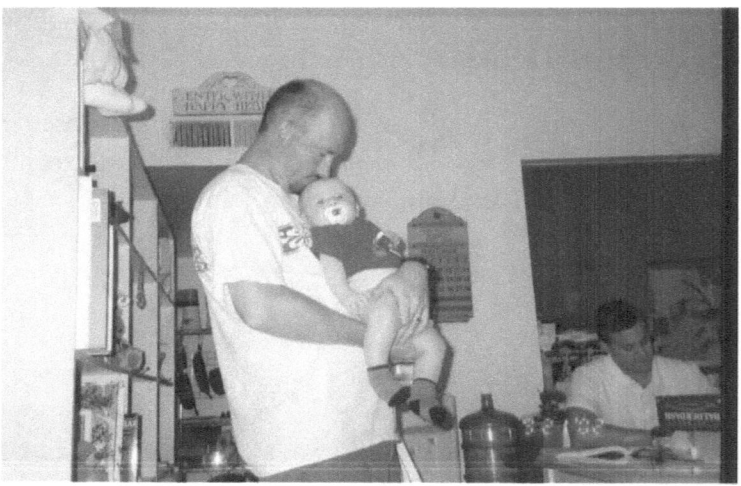

September 18: Even though Jake doesn't sleep through the night consistently, I'm not exhausted at work. But I do often crash in the evenings in front of the TV, especially if Jake's sleeping on me. This week, Jake has been enjoying 3 a.m. feedings. Today I send a FedEx care package to Grandma and Gramps at the hospital.

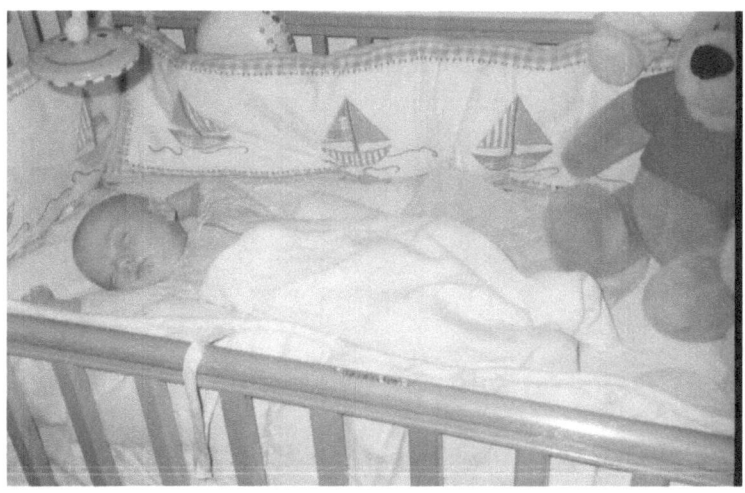

September 23: Today Auntie Caroline turns 29! We sent her gift last week.

A typical Jake day at 14 weeks:

3 a.m.	Nurses (if he wakes up crying)
7 a.m.	Nurses
8-10 a.m. (or longer)	Morning nap in bouncy seat
10:30-noon	Has 5 oz bottle (can take awhile to get interested)
Noon	Plays with Daddy
2 p.m.	Goes to school with Scott (he coaches until 3:30 p.m.)
4-6 p.m.	Afternoon nap in swing
6:30 p.m.	Nurses, then plays
10:30 p.m.	Nurses, then to bed

September 24: Jake will hold a toy or rattle now and put it in his mouth. Today I begin typing my manuscript: *The Genesis of Jake.*

September 25: Jake is **so** cute with smiling and giggling. Every time is like a gift—a little bit of heaven. And I'm sure you can imagine that he gets a lot of positive reinforcement.

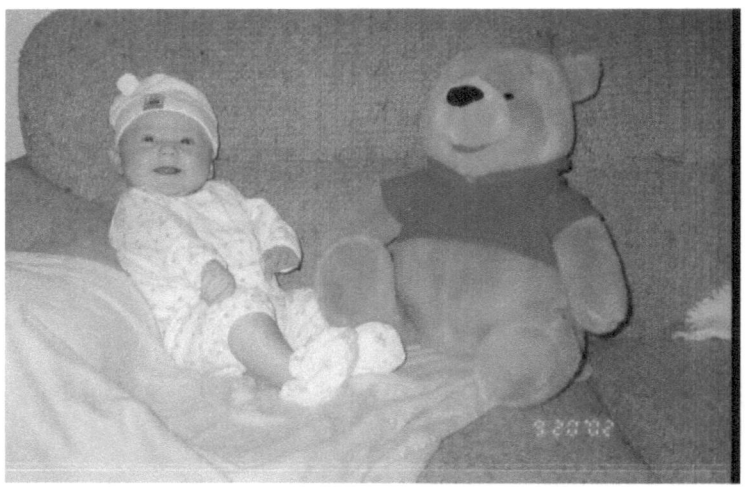

September 26: It's so unbelievably hot. Scott takes Jake to the fourth Baby & Me Lapsit at the Mesa Library today. He reports that Jake smiles and is more active. Scott also says, "It's sad that it's the last one". It's so nice that he took him for three weeks. Jake drools some now, especially when he's "eating fists", which he loves to do.

September 27: Tonight is Jake's third Diamondbacks game! The D'backs' Magic Number is 1, in order to clinch the division again.

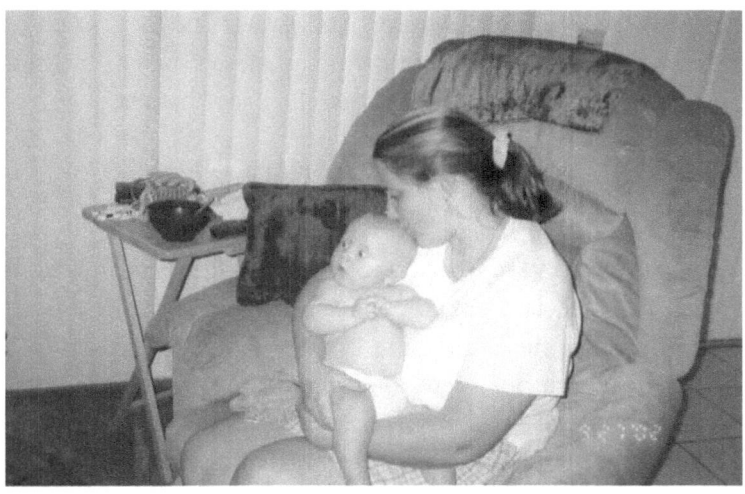

September 28: Jake is 15 weeks old and is now trying to sit up from a slight reclining position, trying to lean forward. He slept 7½ hours last night, which is a recent record. He was very tired after the game. Although he had a short nap after nursing, he was awake most of the game. We were very lucky to be offered a five-pack of Infiniti level seats this season. This is one of the only areas in BOB where I would feel comfortable nursing. Today Scott, Jake and I pick out Scott's new "birthday suit" together at Macy's.

September 29: Jake is 15½ lbs now on our home scale. Gramps flies home from NYC today. The worst of his nightmare is over, but Grandma is driving home alone, so hers will not end quite so soon.

September 30: Overnight, the weather changes to cool. Today we finally break out the video camera. Can you believe it took us 3½ months?! We're lucky Grandma took lots of videos of Jake's first two months before they left on their trip back east.

October 2: Grandma arrives home from NYC (aka "Mordor") today. Jake "talks" a lot now. In fact, he will "converse" with us for several minutes, in "oohs" and "ohs". It's really cute. He smiles easily and giggles, especially with his best buddy: **HIS DADDY**. This evening Jake and I attend a La Leche League meeting at Mesa General Hospital. It's our first time and it's kind of fun to see the other babies.

October 3: Now it's downright cold. Our D'backs are down 0-2 in the opening NL playoff series.

October 4: It's one year since Jake "began" with a swimmer and an egg. Today is Scott's last day of FMLA leave. Four weeks was what he requested, although he could take up to 12 weeks unpaid by law. I think he's a little sad, but these four weeks have forged a tighter bond between him and the little guy. Jake turns to the sound of his voice and, if he's fussy, his mood changes instantly upon hearing Scott.

October 5: Jake is 16 weeks old. To celebrate my 33rd birthday, Scott and I host Dice Game #3. Grandma helps take care of Jake during the party. We have 21 people, so it's one of the largest dice games we've ever played in.

October 6: Scott did such a great job with planning my party, food and cleaning up! Today Jake, Scott and I visit Oktoberfest at the Tempe Town Lake. Jake does really well with Kathy at our softball game.

October 7: Turns out Kathy was in the beginning stages of labor when she was watching Jake last night! Abryanna is born today. Today is Jake's first day "out of the house". Of course we've always taken him places, starting with his first week…all those trips to the lab and back to the doctor! He's going to Grandma's on Mondays and Thursdays, and Alisa's on Tuesdays and Wednesdays. Scott picks him up and we alternate dropping off. Scott left with Jake at 6:45 a.m. and he will pick him up by 4 p.m. Grandma's arsenal is stocked: vibrating chair, swing, 2 bottles plus frozen milk, playpen, diapers, wipes, plus all of mine & Heidi's books and toys! And she bought a stroller yesterday, as well. It's sure a big schedule change for Jakie today…very quiet this morning as I get ready for work.

October 8: Today I drop Jake at Alisa's. It was so kind of her and Jason to make this commitment to watch Jake for a few months, while he's still so young. They didn't want us to have to worry about finding a daycare center yet. Of course we insisted on paying her a fair wage for her time, comparable to the market cost of day care in our area which is $25-35 per day for infants under the age of one.

October 9: I travel to Long Beach this morning, pump and all. The heavy security screening since 9/11 adds additional stress to my day, because I'm chosen for a random check at the gate. The four security screeners in Terminal 4 set forth to entirely dismantle my pump equipment, supplies and icebag. None of them has ever actually seen a breast pump apparatus and it would be humorous in a Keystone-Cop-type of way if it wasn't so intrusive and embarrassing. Thank goodness I've just come from home, so there is no actual milk in the bag yet. I'm truly near tears when I'm told they have no latex gloves. This is crazy! All my bottles and pump parts, clean and sterilized, will now need to be rewashed before I can pump at the Long Beach Marriott, because their grubby hands have pawed through every item. I'm thankful for: (a) a nice restroom at the hotel, where I can carefully wash all my equipment and (b) the opportunity to comfortably pump at Caroline's later in the afternoon. Today Scott has to drop off and pick up Jake, plus be on baby duty all evening. This makes for a long, tiring day for him when he's on his feet all day. I'm so glad to have the opportunity to visit with Caroline and Arnold for a few hours before my plane leaves. I tour their cute new townhouse and they treat me to a lovely birthday dinner in downtown Orange.

October 10: I'm 33 today. I don't really care. I'm just glad we are young enough to have a family and we certainly hope to get pregnant again before I'm 35 and in a higher risk class. I endure six straight hours of meetings at work and a very busy day. Scott gives me a beautiful opal bracelet, Spongebob Squarepants lounge pants and a book.

Jake gives me the Beauty & the Beast DVD for us to watch together. Scott and I enjoy a peaceful evening at the Melting Pot.

October 11: Today I bathe Jake for the first time in weeks, because Scott's been doing it while I'm at work. It's fun!

October 12: Jake's now 17 weeks and nearly 4 months old. He takes his 3rd out-of-town trip, his 2nd trip to Payson. We stay at Heidi and Bill's condo Friday night and come back Saturday evening. This was the first week he could giggle "for real", out loud. We can tickle him and make him laugh. Jake really enjoys holding things and putting them in his mouth.

October 13: Tonight is my birthday dinner with Scott's family, at Mary's. Jake weighs 16-6 on the BestFed scale and is 25" (home measurement).

October 14: I go to Grandma's at lunchtime to feed Jakie! I haven't been feeding him as often at lunch, with Scott back at work. Sometimes Scott would bring him and my lunch to me and we'd visit and nurse in the shade at the Pointe resort. Tonight I experience the strangest feeling...I know Jake has grown and is so big, but watching Grandma's video of his first two months, I was blown away by how small he was and how much he has changed, in such a short life!

October 15: Today Jake is four months into the world! I am so tired today that I have to leave work early. We will implement "bottle night" 2 times per week, instead of just on Saturday nights.

October 16: It takes me an hour to get to work after I leave home, when I drop Jake off at Alisa's. We always like to chat and sometimes I nurse him one last time. Luckily, it's all freeway from their house to work.

October 17: Our weather is really cooling off nicely. It's 75-80° now. I've been experiencing an itching problem since last week. My nurse says it's probably a yeast infection—apparently the body produces no estrogen when breastfeeding, so they are more likely to occur.

October 18: The three of us go to Jake's 4-month doctor's appointment today. It's very nice to go as a family. Jake cries when he gets his shots but cheers up when Daddy makes him smile and giggle, as usual.

October 19: Jake is 18 weeks old today—it's getting hard to count the weeks now, so I guess it's time to switch to months! Jake is quite a traveler and usually does okay in the carseat. He goes on all sorts of errands this weekend…helps keep me busy while Heidi and Bill moved in with Grandma and Gramps, parties at Jason and Alisa's, goes to stores with Daddy, visits Heidi and Bill's new house under construction and ends the weekend with a trip to the softball field.

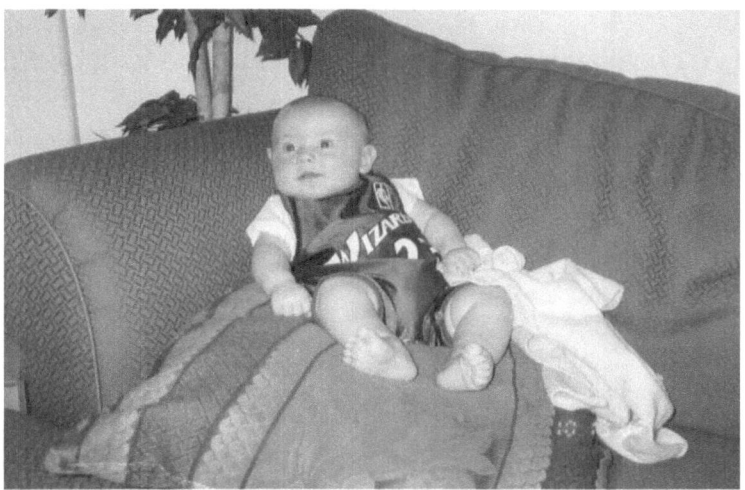

October 20: What a sweet baby. I love him so much! We have such nice snuggles. Scott says he falls asleep on me exclusively. But Daddy can make him laugh **on demand**, especially in the last few weeks. He still loves taking a bath—just once a week. Our co-ed softball season draws to a close this evening and we have our playoff game next week.

October 22: I receive a stock option package today, provided I'm still with OmniMount in 2005! WOW! I notice Jake eats less often and I wonder if he's getting enough breastmilk and if he's near the "average". I'm still tracking every feeding as a tool. Over the last five days, I estimate he's getting 20 oz/day. That's interesting because the "average" intake for 4-6 months is 31 oz/day and "average" intake for a baby weighing 16 lbs is 43 oz/day. Hmmm.... We feed on demand, so I guess it doesn't really matter.

October 23: Today Alisa confirms, "I'm yours until Christmas". She doesn't say "only", but we understand what she means and that her time alone with her own preschoolers is precious. We so appreciate the time she has given up for us. What a huge sacrifice she has made to take Jake in this crucial developmental stage. We need to begin looking for alternate daycare arrangements.

October 24: Grandma reports that Jake sits up and leans over from a semi-recline position. Scott confirms that he's also seen this recently. We take Jake to the doctor today because he's had a cough for five days and now it's more in his chest, sounding congested. She says it's still okay. He still weighs 16-8. Grandma offers to take Jake four days per week in January if necessary because she doesn't want him to have to go to a stranger.

October 25: We take the cute "pumpkin picture" at Fiesta Mall today!

October 27: Jake often reaches and grabs us now. He can hold toys well. I'm having serious negotiations with Scott about hiring a maid.

October 28: Grandma loves her new saucer that we got last Friday. She reports that Jake enjoys it!

October 29: Jake rolls over on the waterbed this morning as I'm getting ready for work. I don't witness the roll, but I find him on his on his back after I put him on his tummy. The real thing will be soon!

October 31: Jake's first Halloween! He wears his pumpkin costume for the occasion, although it's a bit warm. He helps us hand out candy.

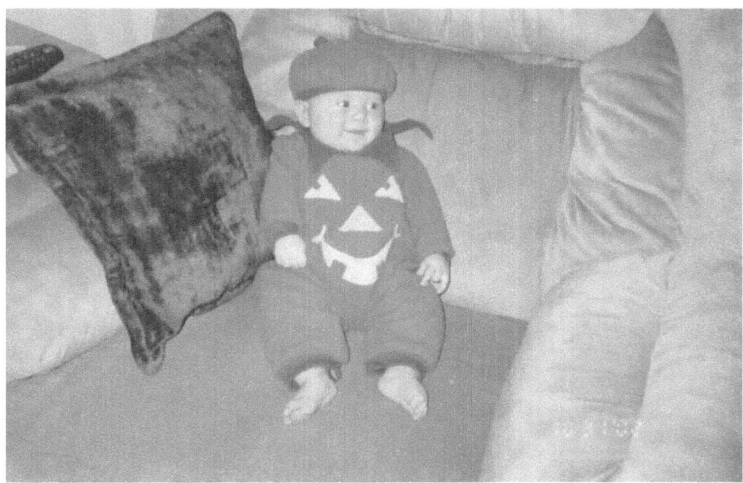

November 1: I catch Jake playing with his toes and feet this morning! He looks so big to me now! Today is a big day: our first professional housecleaning.

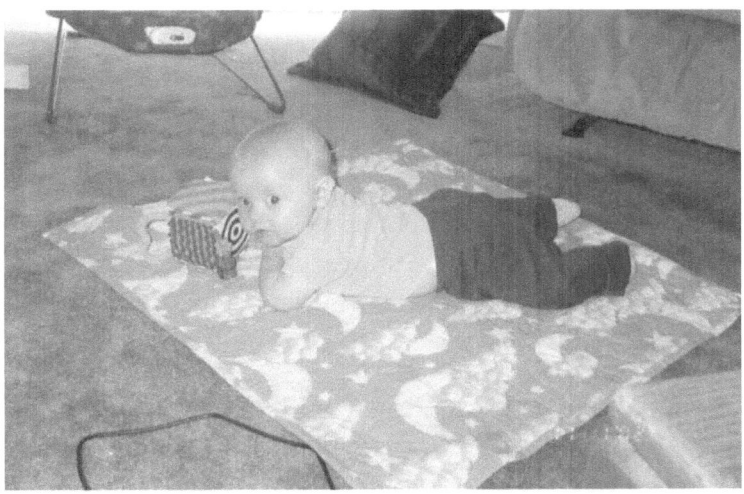

November 2: Jake is 20 weeks old now. I notice some "multitasking" this weekend. Jake has my finger in his hand, in his mouth and his other hand playing with his foot! This from someone who couldn't eat while passing gas/pooping. Ha.

November 3: Jake still enjoys his baths and is so cute! Tonight Scott and I are very sick and we're not sure if we have food poisoning or a 24-hour flu.

November 4: Breastfeeding is scary today since my sickness might be passed in my milk? I don't know but I accept the small risk.

November 5: For the last three nights, Jake has slept over eight hours each night! Go Jake! Tonight, we have dinner at Oregano's with Aunt Heidi, Uncle Bill, Grandma, Gramps, Marilyn, Dave, Cheryl and Tim. Fun!

November 6: Uh-oh. We find out that Heidi, Bill, Grandma, Cheryl and Tim all got sick. Jake is spared—or he's the carrier. Tonight is Jake's first Phoenix Suns game! We beat the Atlanta Hawks. Jake did great and was awake nearly all of the game.

November 7: I stay home with Jake today, so Grandma can rest and feel better. I do work about two hours from home.

November 8: My illness ended up pushing me over a long plateau. Now I'm down 40 lbs since Jake's birthday. I have 22 left to go.

November 9: Jake is 21 weeks old now. I can't believe we have a baby who will be five months old next week! At the Fall Festival at BTW tonight, everyone who sees Jake says how cute and precious he is. See, we're not just biased!

November 10: Jake weighs 18 lbs on our home scale, with clothes. He likes to try to eat his feet—what flexibility! He makes goo-goo gurgly noises with saliva and has lots of drool.

November 11: I'm no longer wearing any nursing pads because I realized I never leak anymore. Gabriele, president of the official Jake Eggen Italian fan club, who made the mistake of being interested in Jake's pictures so now receives them regularly, says of Jake at Halloween: "he is the epitome of placidness". We bought Jake's first solid food this weekend, so tonight I assembled the high chair!

November 12: Jake loves to play with his feet while he's on the changing table. Sometimes he tries to put them in his mouth.

November 13: You know what's weird? That my body has been Jake's **sole** source of nourishment for over 13 months! Alisa said Jake rolled over today, at their house. There was a very slight incline in his favor, but Daddy concurred that it was a real roll. Alisa encouraged Jake with a stuffed animal and got it on video for us.

November 15: Five months old! Jake is so sweet. He's quite active now and so alert. He loves to grab things and put them in his mouth. He weighs 17 lbs, 10 oz (BestFed scale, without clothes) and is approx 26 inches. Today we all participated in a five-mile walk for Making Strides for Breast Cancer, with Jason, Alisa, Harv, Norma, Lauren and Kayden. Jake went along in the stroller and did great! He's a very smiley and happy baby. There have been **lots** of giggles with Daddy and with Grandma lately—and just a few with Mom. ☺

November 17: Today, I caught Jake in the swing, trying to get his foot in his mouth. He can't get the same leverage and stretch as on the changing table! (plus jammie feet are slippery work) Jake is now experimenting with lots of noises: "talking", squeals, giggles, songs and "mamum", which I of course especially appreciate because of what it sounds like!

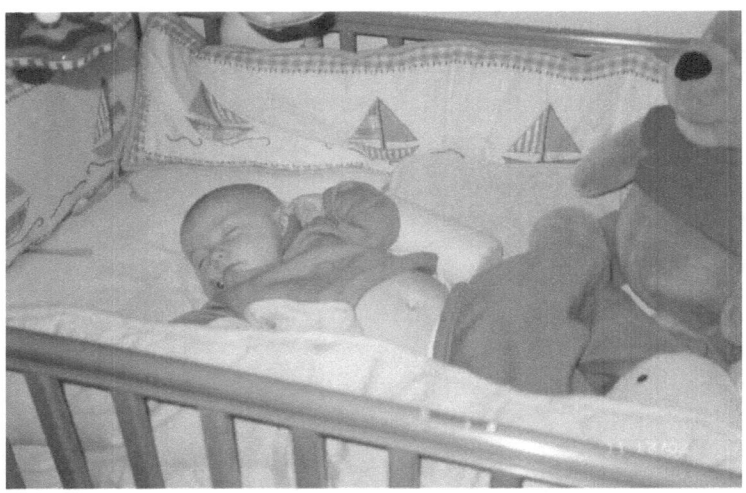

November 18: Scott and I celebrate our 2-year wedding anniversary! This year's theme is "cotton", so Scott presents me with an ingenious frame covered in cotton balls. I also stick to the cotton theme with matching ASU sweatshirts for him and Jake, plus an ASU cap and pajamas for Jake "dreaming of being an ASU star". I'm such a good sport! Anyway, it's hard to believe that it's already been two years! Last year I was pregnant when we went to the Marquesa. It seems like yesterday. Sean babysits so we can go to dinner at the Seafood Market, recently relocated to the old Red Robin of our first date fame. Jake was so unhappy this evening. He cried and screamed inconsolably from 6-6:30 p.m., threatening to spoil our evening out. Scott was able to get him to sleep when I gave up. This is rare for Jake. It's very possible that he's teething, though.

November 19: Alisa only has five more weeks (10 actual days) left to watch Jake, if it's only 'til Christmas. Today starts her 7th week.

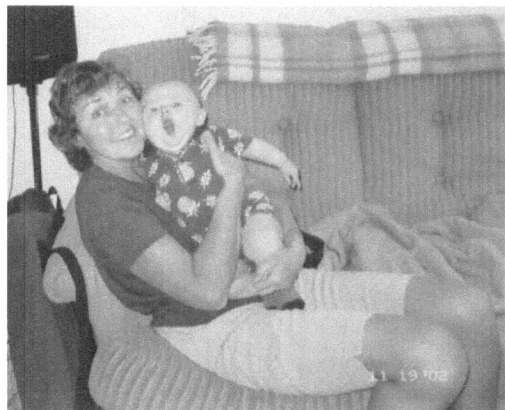

November 20: At 7 a.m., Jake enjoys sitting in the "big chair" (our recliner) and watching *Teletubbies*, *Caillou* and the beginning of *Sesame Street* (8 a.m.) before we leave for Alisa's.

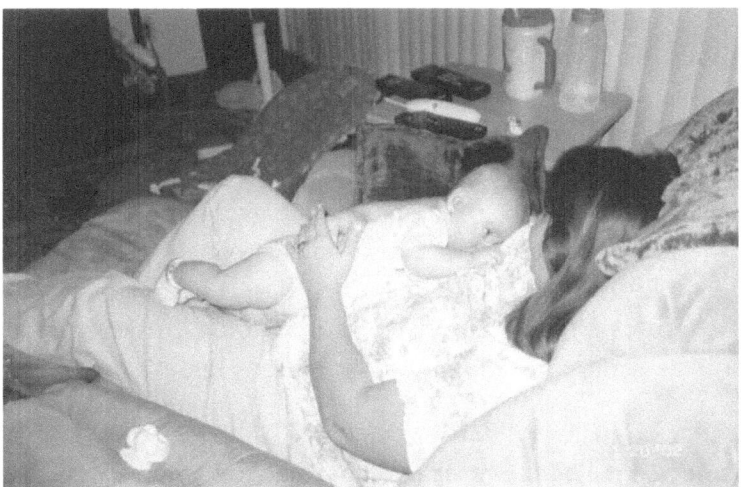

November 22: This has been another (rare) week of Jake sleeping through the night! I enjoy my Fridays with Jake so much! I worked about five hours today since he took such good naps. That was out-

standing because I'm behind schedule on certain projects, including one that needs to be in place by January 1.

November 23: Jake is 23 weeks old. To Shari's for a softball BBQ.

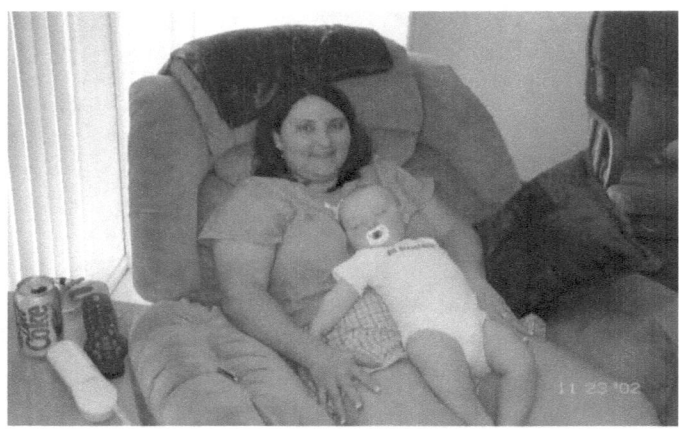

November 24: I get to hang out with Jake all weekend! Our "Sunday Morning Snuggle" is the best—all three of us in the waterbed. Sometimes I think about the fact that Jake is the only child who will get this snuggle to himself. Today, Scott and I look at a lakefront house in Dobson Ranch. We want to upgrade to a bigger house (five bedroom?) before or shortly following the next baby, because we will have outgrown our little three bedroom house. The lakefront house has just three bedrooms, plus an office, workroom and a gorgeous deck, so it may still be a bit too tight. I get **so many giggles** with peek-a-boo tonight!

November 25: Today we find out Holly is pregnant, due June 9, 2003. This will be Holly and Marc's fourth, and last, baby. Today I really missed Jake. I love our "3-day-weekends" together.

November 26: Jake loves to look around in the car when we are driving to Alisa's in the morning. He can sit up with help now, but will flop over if he's alone. Lauren and Kayden are so sweet with Jake.

November 27: Today I'm working a ½ day so I can pick up Honey Bear's and I was able to move up my nail appointment from Friday. It's the day before Thanksgiving and our big Pershall Family Reunion is tomorrow in Chandler. Our family starts arriving this evening and Jake meets (Great-)Uncle Bob, Aunt Emily, Uncle Gene, and Aunts Margaret, Vera and Patty. He's great.

November 28: 90 people at the reunion today! We are there from noon to 5 p.m. It's very fun and goes better food-wise than we had expected. All the cousins really pitched in and there's a lot of food left over that someone takes to a women's shelter. Jake's really good all day and naps there in his stroller. Later we have dinner #2 with Uncle Doug, Aunt Mary and Brad at Mimi's, coming home for pie and to watch *Lord of the Rings*, also with Grandma and Gramps.

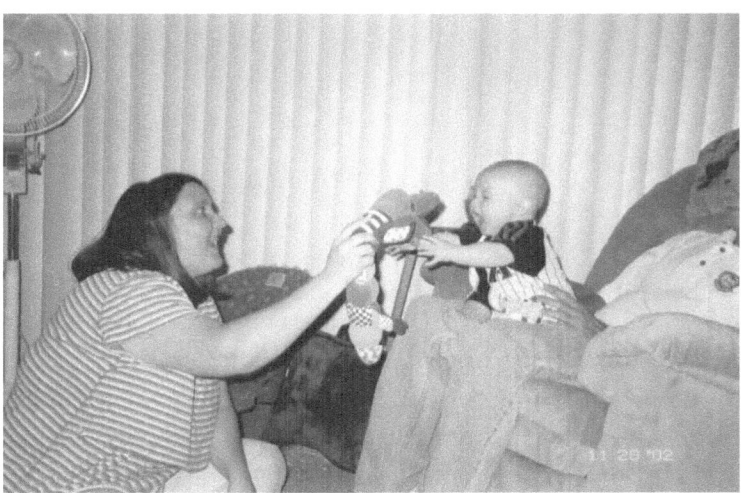

November 29: Jake is so alert and active, grabbing things. He sits with just a little assistance, if he's at the right angle (falls over if not).

December 1: At 5½ months, Jake sits alone, with only a "spotter".

December 2: I'm very low on frozen breastmilk. In fact, I've taken an inventory. We have 3 bags of 4 oz each and 8 bags of 5 oz each. Grandma has 2 bags and Alisa has 2 or 3 bags. Wow! It certainly was depleted quickly. Speaking of quickly, it's wild how quickly Jake catches on to how toys work, like touching them and kicking them, after only one demonstration of how it works! He does it immediately—so smart!

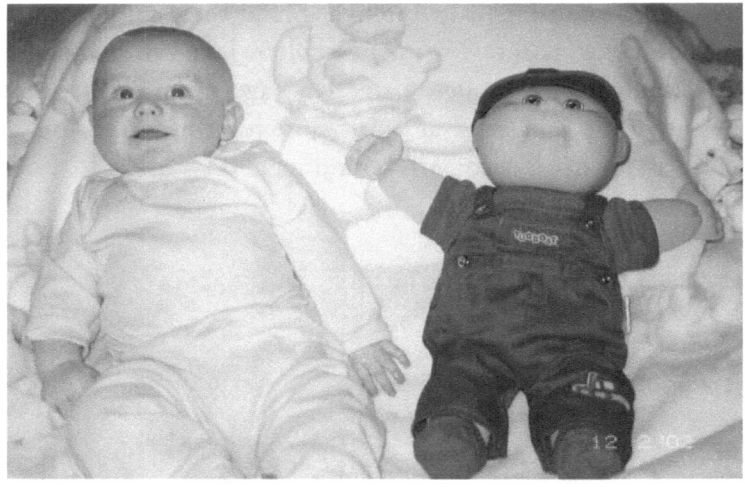

December 3: Last night I installed the play mirror in Jake's crib and I encouraged him to investigate it and roll towards it. He's a slow roller as opposed to a high roller. I decided it's time to take away his sleep positioner, which he has been sleeping in since we brought him home from the hospital. It's designed to encourage babies to sleep on their backs, since current scientific theory says SIDS is less common if babies sleep on their backs—the slogan of the year is "Back to Sleep"....

Today I got my engagement/wedding rings off for the first time in nearly one year! Gave 'em a darn good cleaning. My fingers were so swollen during the pregnancy.

December 4: Tonight is our first Infant Massage class at BestFed. We're in the class with only one other family and Jake is very good. He weighs 18-1 with no clothes now.

December 5: Last night Jake slept through the night again, which we define by "until 5 a.m. or later". In fact, this is becoming more regular and he probably sleeps through the night 8 out of 10 nights now.... But he is SO hungry when he wakes up!

December 6: I feel Jake's very first tooth poking through his bottom gum today. Tonight, Jake enjoys his 2nd Suns game!

December 7: I have been reading *Prodigal Summer* since August, usually when I'm "hooked up" to my breast pump. Today I finish it, finally! I can't believe this is the first book I've managed to finish since Jake was born. It's a great book.

December 8: Jake bites when nursing now! Twice today! OUCH! I told him "NO!" and I think I scared him. Today is his first bath where he's very curious to look around and he even tries to reach a towel laying near his tub, by sitting up. So cute! We probably don't have many more baths in the small tub on the kitchen counter, as he's getting pretty big for it now.

December 10: Occasional biting during nursing.... This seems to happen most often when he's finished because he tightens and turns. Also happens when he's impatient because there's not enough milk right away...maybe the letdown is slow sometimes?

December 12: Grandma reports that Jake really enjoys looking at cars when they are on a walk in the stroller. She says he is very sweet!

December 14: Scott and I are feeling very rushed, trying to finish our Christmas shopping. Jake goes with us to Scott's BTW Christmas party at the old Duck & Decanter lake.

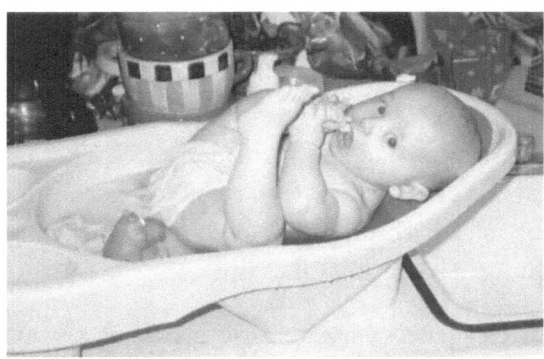

December 15: Jake is *SIX MONTHS OLD* already! Today is another fun bath, although Jake loves to sit up and now he's getting too close for comfort to bumping his head on the underside of the kitchen cabinet. He's busy reaching for the cookie jar and the pitcher. Today, because he loves to touch things, he was absolutely MESMERIZED by the water pouring from the pitcher, trying to touch it and hold it. He just stared at it, with a hint of a smile. He still naps about 1½ hours in the morning and at least another 1-2 hours in the afternoon. Usually, around 8-9 p.m., he takes another nap in his swing. BIG DAY TODAY: Jake eats his first food other than breastmilk…rice cereal. He did not like it one bit. I don't think I'll ever forget that grimace. We had a little "half-birthday" party for our "little halfling". Tonight is also Doug and Ellie's (real) birthday party.

December 16: I feel behind at work and feel that four days a week in the office isn't enough. I bring work home on Fridays but I don't get to it nearly often enough and I'm feeling bad about it. But I cherish every single minute with Jake Friday through Sunday!!

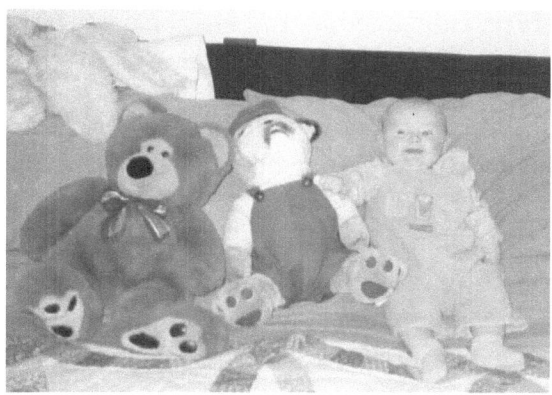

December 17: I take the morning off today to take Jake to his six month doctor's appointment. She says everything looks good! Jake has his six-month shots, which aren't too bad—just brief crying. She gives us a prescription for iron/vitamin drops. Now his next appointment is at 9 months (3/17/03).

December 18: Today is Jake's last day at Alisa's. Maybe we can still have some prearranged play dates, though! What a wonderful gift she gave Jake: her time.

December 19: The sound of Jake laughing (giggling) is the best sound in the entire world. ☺

December 20: Neal (finally) graduates from ASU today. Jake naps through the second half. Scott and I notice today that a second tooth is trying to come in! It's right next to the first one on the bottom.

December 21: Today is our 2nd try at feeding Jake cereal. He's still not very happy about it and even gagged a little. Instead of mixing it with breastmilk, we tried using formula this time. I finally broke out the sample from the hospital. Jake and I go to Chandler Mall later to finish Christmas shopping while Daddy gets us a Christmas tree (better late than never, I say). We chose a potted version this year, so we can plant it. It's just four feet tall. Grandma and Heidi babysit Jake tonight while Scott and I go to the Suns game, with 9th row seats!

December 22: I'm plotting how we'll manage when I am in Las Vegas for two days January 6-7 at the credit meeting. We're trying a new veggie or fruit every fifth day, so that's a small supplemental food source. Since we are so low on frozen milk, I think we'll need to plan on using some formula, testing it over the next two weeks to make sure he has no adverse reaction. I counted how many bottles Scott will need while I'm gone: *seven.* Unless I can freeze any extra over my Christmas break, we'll definitely be short. I do plan on pumping in Las Vegas, if I'm sure I'll have a way of keeping the milk chilled. I don't want to go to all the trouble, just to have to dump it later.

December 23: Scott is home with Jake until January 5th!

December 24: Jake's first Christmas Eve, the evening spent out at Marc and Holly's. This year, we have the littlest Eggen there. Scott says, "It's sad that he's not going to be this size forever." I understand completely because he is so sweet at this age. Jake gets to try green beans today for the first time and they are not quite as undesirable as cereal. All our first samples of fruits and vegetables are from the game at my baby shower!

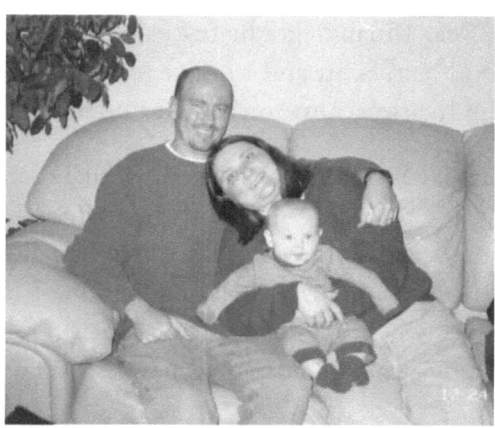

December 25: Christmas falls on a Wednesday this year, the worst possible day. Garret, however, has decided to make 12/26 and 12/27 both company-paid holidays as well this year! Yeah! Jake's first Christmas is a busy one: we're gone from 9:20 a.m. until 10:10 p.m., but it's a very fun day. First to Grandpa's for breakfast, then to Grandma's and then on to Uncle Duane's. Jake and I both sleep in Mackenzie's play room. We're exhausted by the end of the day!

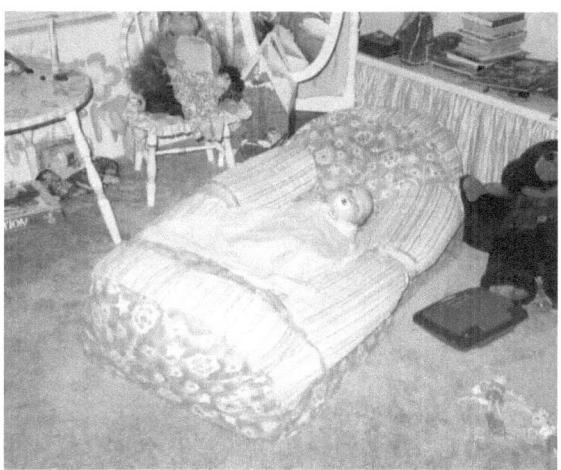

December 26: Today, I will go nowhere and just recuperate! My milk seems low. My last two pumping sessions have resulted in just 1 oz from each side.... Formula is necessary for the first time today. Thankfully, Jake doesn't mind it at all, or really even seem to notice the difference. We have just one bag of frozen milk remaining.

December 28: Jake is so observant and really reaches out for things now. He loves his saucer and his "key ring" toy that Daddy/Santa got him. Jake is so smiley.

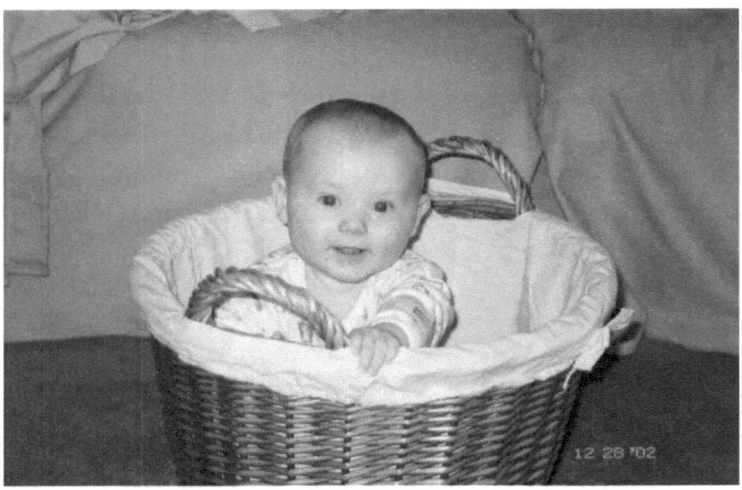

December 29: I'm so selfish—this is my fifth day off and I still don't want to go back to work tomorrow. I love being home with Scott and Jake. Jake sits alone now, but falls over sometimes.

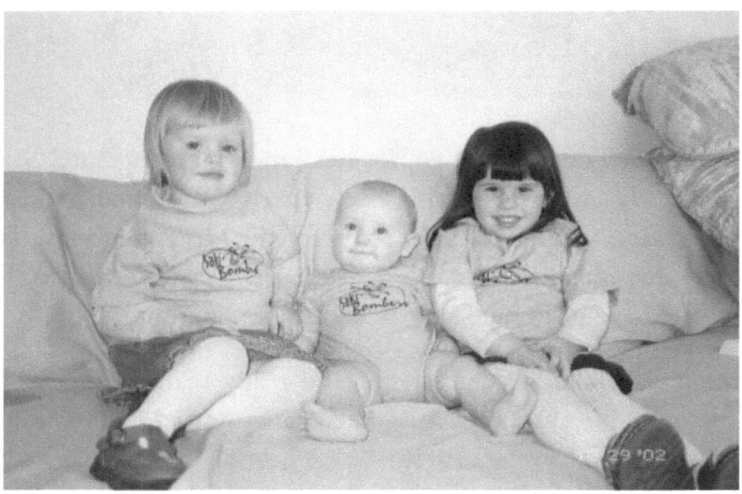

December 30: Jake is rounding to 19 lbs on our home scale now, with clothes, so he's probably 18½. He's finally getting some hair!

December 31: It's disappointing now when I pump at work. I used to pump 5 oz regularly (total) and now I'm lucky to get 2½. ☹ I'm glad I broke down and opened the formula so Jake wouldn't starve! We'll just nurse as long as there's milk…. Jake spends his first New Year's Eve at Zoo Lights with Mama, Daddy and Jason, Alisa, Kayden and Lauren. Chilly, but so fun!

January 1, 2003: My New Year's thoughts…

- Enjoy every minute!

- Never take Scott for granted! (it's unbelievable how much he does)

- Jake will never be 6½ – 18½ months again. Spend as much time together as we can!

- This year is the "sister trip" with Heidi! (every two years we go)

- Steph's graduation from law school—May 2003!

- Do we want to try for Baby #2? (then they will be 2+ years apart)

- If so, I'd like Jake's "baby fat" off first. I've got a ways to go….

- Spend time with Mom & Dad every week; continue walking Dad.

- Do something just for me every week.

- At work, focus on helping others succeed.

- Get a different viewpoint if things look difficult or stuck—remember that just one small change can make a big difference.

- Be proud! In 2001, only 32.5% of new moms nursed until their baby was six months old (according to survey by Ross Products—this is the highest rate since they started the survey in 1954). I breastfed Jake exclusively for his first six months. ☺

January 5: Today we arrive home from our trip to Sedona. We had so much fun with Jake. This morning before we left we took a family bath with bath bubbles, in the jacuzzi! That was one slippery baby. Yesterday we did what we swore we WOULDN'T do: buy a timeshare! This one was repossessed, so it was paid down some. I can't believe we actually signed the contract. But it does seem like a good investment and will offer some really nice vacation opportunities, when we trade it through the exchange book. Can I tell you how ANGRY I was when they said Jake couldn't come with us into the timeshare presentation and that he had to stay with the on-site babysitter?! I was livid and in tears. Don't ever tell me my baby can't be with me. That was our first time leaving Jake with a stranger and it was horrible.

January 8: Home from another trip today (back-to-back trips). I was in Las Vegas, with Claudia, at the national credit meeting. This was my first overnight stay without Jake! I pumped a lot! In fact, I arrived home with about 17 oz of milk! (trying desperately to keep it cool because I couldn't refreeze my ice pack) I missed Jake and Scott and our home very much!...Today Jake tries bananas (banana baby food smells very strange). We've also sampled green beans, rice cereal, oat cereal (both are yuck), applesauce and peaches. Jake has swallowed a fair amount of peaches and bananas.

January 11: Jake is very giggly and happy. He loves to sit and play now, especially with his Discovery Snail, a gift from my cousin, Susan. He sits in the Boppy for support or plays in his saucer. He reaches and grabs at everything now: people's hair, clothes, our long hanging plant in the kitchen. His generally-followed eating habits at this stage:

7 a.m.	Nurses
11 a.m.	Bottle of formula
2 p.m.	Bottle of formula (at work, I'm pumping at 1 p.m. only)
6-7 p.m.	Might have a bit of baby food, nurses, plus a formula bottle or pumped milk bottle if he's still hungry

| 8-9 p.m. | Pumped milk bottle |
| 10-11 p.m. | Nurses, then to bed (most nights he's sleeping through!) |

January 15: Jake is seven months old! "Big Jake", taking a few liberties with the John Wayne reference here, weighs in at 19½ lbs and when I stand him up against his Pooh growth chart taped on the wall, it looks like he's 28 inches now. It's strange but I've noticed that even though I seem to not be producing as much breast milk now, there actually may be some that just hasn't "let down" yet. Sometimes I'm surprised at the end of a pumping session to have more coming when I would otherwise be ready to turn the pump off.

January 17: I still have Fridays at home and I'm grateful. I don't know if I can rationalize it forever. I'm swamped at work and this gives me fewer hours in the week to get it all done. I don't get much done at home on Fridays. Here is a very fun thing: hearing, and watching, Jake laugh and laugh at Scott's "Donald Duck" voice and other silly noises. We may not get out much but this is some pretty darn good entertainment!…Jake rolls over in his swing today! This is bad news, but we'll just have to start buckling him in. He also rolls over at will. For the first time, I have found him on his tummy in his crib this week. He first did this a few weeks ago but this week he's turning over more regularly…. Since he's grown, he's now on the 2nd notch in his saucer, which is height-adjustable with 3 levels. He plays on the floor now, just as often as he plays in his saucer. Sometimes we use the Boppy for him to sit in so he doesn't fall, but he sits very well on his own now. He is intrigued by small things and loves to investigate them: the button on the Björn, the antennae on the Discovery Snail.

January 23: Very scary moment for Scott today: Jake fell out of the swing! We've been careful to buckle him in, since he exhibited his new turning-over-in-the-swing skills, but today Uncle Sean had laid him in it after his sleepy bottle…and didn't realize the strap was necessary…. Jake's eating food very well now. It took a full month and lots of patience on Gramps' part…. This has been a very stressful week for me at work, trying to deal with banking issues, vendor issues, department staffing issues, the year-end audit hanging over me, and to top it off I've been given a raise…and my anxiety level has been raised proportionately.

January 24: We are mobile! Today Jake makes his first crawling motion…backward! It's really more creeping, than crawling. He travels 2-3 feet at Grandma's and demonstrates for his parents later at home. At 7 months and 9 days, Jake is officially "on the move"! It's really time to safety-proof. It's now or never.

February 1: Aunt Heidi and Uncle Bill spend their first night in their brand new house! We all help move them in today: Grandma, Gramps, Grandpa, Steve, Sean, Mama, Daddy and Jake, who is an excellent supervisor! Before we started filling the moving truck, we mourned the lives of the space shuttle Columbia astronauts who died this morning. The shuttle exploded upon re-entry over Texas, 17 years and 4 days after we watched the Challenger blow up on live TV.

…At 7½ months old, Jake's food intake is 50% formula, 30% solid food and just 20% breast milk. My milk production is low and Jake is very impatient if there's not "enough" or if it's not letting down fast enough for him. This is so frustrating for both of us. As such, formula supplements have become absolutely mandatory. His most recently added solid foods are carrots and rice cereal mixed with peach apple. Unfortunately, all the solids have led to his first bouts of constipation and crying fits. His bowel movements are more solid now…. Jake is not as unhappy playing on his tummy now, since he can lift his tummy slightly off the floor!

February 2: Jake enjoys his first jar of prunes today. We hope it helps his constipation. He's really funny when he's nursing now. On the left side, he lies normally, but on the right side, he's quite wiggly. He ends up moving all around, after starting in the cradle position, ending up between my legs on his tummy. He wants to crawl but he's still learning the "concepts"!

February 4: We must have overdone it on the prunes! After the small jar on Sunday, we added a half jar on Monday. Lo and behold, Jake has had about 10 messy diapers over the last two days! In fact it was so bad that Grandma had to give him a bath today. Let it be a lesson that prunes are effective for small tummies in small portions.... How long has it been that he's been sleeping through the night? A month? More? It's very odd how quickly a person forgets, especially on such an important topic like sleep, so crucial to one's coherence and mental health! Tonight is a family walk at Grandpa's, then we make the 20-mile drive to Heidi and Bill's for a quick visit!

February 7: Jake will be 8 months old next week. We take him to the doctor today because of a deep cough. She's concerned about his wheezing and believes he may have been exposed somehow to the RSV virus. She prescribes a breathing treatment of albuterol sulfate and saline, which we must administer every four hours until his next appointment, in five days! She also thinks he may be developing an ear infection, for which she prescribes liquid amoxicillin. Jake is doing fine, but his cough really sounds bad. His official weigh-in today shows 20 lbs 6 oz!

February 11: Today Jake and I surprise Daddy by sneaking down to Chandler Fashion Center and taking a portrait together to give Daddy as a valentine. This is a BIG project all by myself and I barely have the energy. The pictures turn out so cute. Grandpa meets us at the mall!

February 12: Today is Jake's follow-up doctor's appointment and we are informed that his chest sounds better. Now the breathing treatment is to be given every six hours until our next follow-up appointment. It's discouraging because administering both the amoxicillin and the breathing treatment so many times throughout the day is very challenging. Poor little Jake hates them both.

February 13: I feel like I'm coming down with something now. I'm also feeling very anxious and stressed out about work. Talking with my counselor helps. She reminds me that I don't have to be perfect, just "good enough". That applies to me as an employee, a daughter, a wife and a mom! I need to remember to ask for help when I need it.

February 14: Happy First Valentine's Day to Jake! He's 8 months old tomorrow. After a quick cost/benefit analysis, Scott and I make the decision to end the nursing so I can take an anti-depressant medication I need. My family doctor advised weaning so I can take it. It's scary: even though Jake is truly 90% weaned already, it's so damn final. I hate this so much. There is a really good poem on the grief of weaning in my breastfeeding book and it helps me to read it. Scott and Jake send me flowers at work today and I get lots of gifts!

February 16: Three full days of not nursing and my breasts are full of milk. What to do? My breastfeeding "bible" says it's **okay** to nurse on this medication—that it's not much risk of passing substantial quantities on to the baby. So I'm absolutely torn. I don't think I want to pump and try to continue milk production at this point. I hate this. I'm tempted to just go ahead and nurse, if it's not dangerous for Jake.

February 17: Out of desperation, I make the call for a 2nd opinion. Dr. McN.'s nurse says it's fine to go ahead and nurse and "not to worry"! I nurse Jake tonight for the first time in four days! ☺

February 18: I hate going to work right now and I'm fantasizing about quitting every day! This is a very unusual situation because I really love my job and my company!…"The Jakester" rolls around a lot now but still is unable to crawl forward. He can scoot backwards well. He is eating most baby foods, tolerates sips of water and LOVES Cheerios! He ends up wearing more than he eats, but he does a great job of "sogging" them up to be able to gum them. ☺ Thankfully, Jake continues to sleep through the night and sometimes we even need to wake him if it's Scott's morning to take him to Grandma's house.

February 20: Jake's doctor reports that his lungs are clear now! We now are to do the breathing treatments only as needed. Hallelujah! I've grown weary of all these doctor's appointments, especially because it's 10 miles each way. How ironic that we chose this doctor because the office was so close…and then she moved prior to our first appointment!

February 21: The infrequency of breastfeeding has caught up with my body: I have my first real period in 17 months. ***Strange!*** After 20 years with one, you'd think it would be like riding a bike, but it takes some getting used to, all over again.

March 1: At 8½ months, Jake is cutting his third tooth. This is his first top tooth!

March 5: Jake loves to feed himself now: Cheerios, crackers and last night he tried pork and beans, which were apparently very slippery. He's really trying to stand up and is nearly ready to begin crawling. He can still only move backward or roll and then sit up. He's now getting his fourth tooth, also on top.

March 9: Daddy witnesses Jake crawling forward!

March 12: We have visitors from Illinois! Auntie Stephanie and Erik come for a spring break visit. I ditch work and Aunt Heidi and I join them for lunch at The Farm and for boating on the Tempe Town Lake. It's a beautiful spring day. All of a sudden, at 8¾ months, Jake is crawling all over.

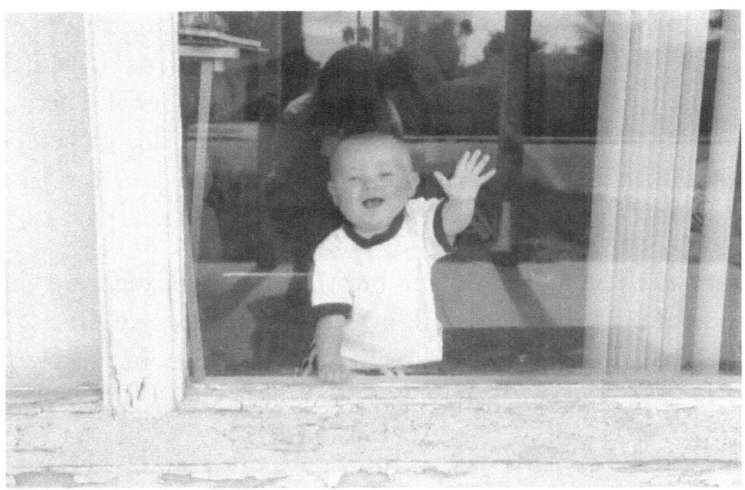

March 17: Our big 9-month-old now wants to try to stand up and BITE EVERYTHING. He's doing more teething now. Sometimes he'll try to bite my legs and of course my fingers. Scott is home with Jake this week on spring break. Thursday through Sunday we are going to Williamsburg, Virginia! We have frequent flier trips that we need to use and a great last minute rate at the timeshare there. It's a little scary trying to pack everything we might possibly need for a baby and a 4-hour flight! Are we certifiably crazy?...President George W. Bush announces tonight that Saddam Hussein has 48 hours to leave Iraq or we will attack him. War is imminent.

March 18: Today is Jake's 9-month check-up at the doctor. This time Daddy gets to take him since he's on vacation. At 21 lbs and 28¼ inches, Jake is in the 50th percentile on height, weight and also head circumference. I've only packed Jake's food for the trip. I'm getting very nervous about his clothes, his stroller and traveling with him! As for Scott, he's nervous about traveling during the war...not to mention this will be his first flight since 9/11/01.

March 19: Now we're packed for Virginia! Adventure awaits!…We attacked Saddam Hussein tonight. I so need a change of scenery so I'm very appreciative to Scott for not insisting we cancel the trip due to the war.

March 23: We have a fabulous time spending 3 nights at Powhatan Plantation. We have only two full days in Virginia, but we're still glad we went. It's Jake's first out-of-state trip and we have a very fun time. Jake crawls FAST now and he can stand up against furniture. He really enjoyed getting into the fireplace! Daddy and Jake have a ball "chasing" each other through the living room and bedroom, on all fours.

March 25: Tonight Jake has his very last serving of thawed breastmilk. It's from the last of the bags I froze in January, as we've been thawing them sparingly. Jake appears to be doing very well on the Similac with iron so I'm happy about that. We really like the single serving packages that make 4 oz of formula. Jake drinks about 16-20 oz of formula every day and he's eating a variety of baby foods 2-3 times per day. He's now at the Stage 3 consistency, which is lumpy. Grandma is enjoying bathing Jake twice a week and often takes him on stroller rides to the neighborhood park. At 9 months and 10 days, Jake is crawling fast, pulling himself up easily to a standing position and, while holding onto furniture, experimenting with taking steps. He is a VERY active and VERY curious child.

March 27: Good meeting today with my counselor, my boss and me. My boss agreed that my list of job responsibilities is "huge", which was a first! We will all work on redesigning my role and planning staffing requirements for my department, so that I can delegate some duties.

March 30: Today I started my 2nd period since ceasing to nurse, on a cycle that's over five weeks, so my body is still adjusting.

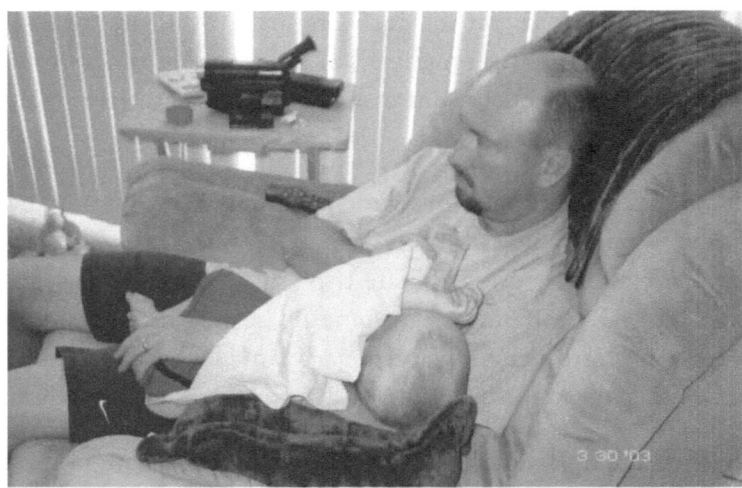

March 31: Today is a good day. I feel productive at work and feel that progress has been made in working to create a better future. Having specific, reachable targets helps me tremendously. Feeling that I am making headway feels really good. Next week I will be starting a standard birth control pill, since it is more effective than the "mini-pill" recommended during nursing.

April 1: Jake is such a **sweetie** at 9½ months! He is happy and is content to play by himself occasionally, for up to 30 minutes! He smiles, giggles, stands up, and picks out his own toys to play with. He continues to nap in the swing, in the late morning and in the late afternoon. He now has six teeth: 2 on the bottom and 4 on the top. He's 21-22 lbs and we are getting ready to move into Size 4 Pampers. He crawls everywhere and loves investigating. He also loves to self-feed, Cheerios especially, although he'll eat anything at this point. The least welcome food option is a potato; maybe it's too bland, or just has an undesirable texture. Jake sleeps 9-10 hours every night, unless his diapers spring a leak and his wet jammies wake him up. He continues to use and love his "paci"-fier and enjoys feeling very small threads and crumbs, rubbing them between his thumb and forefinger.

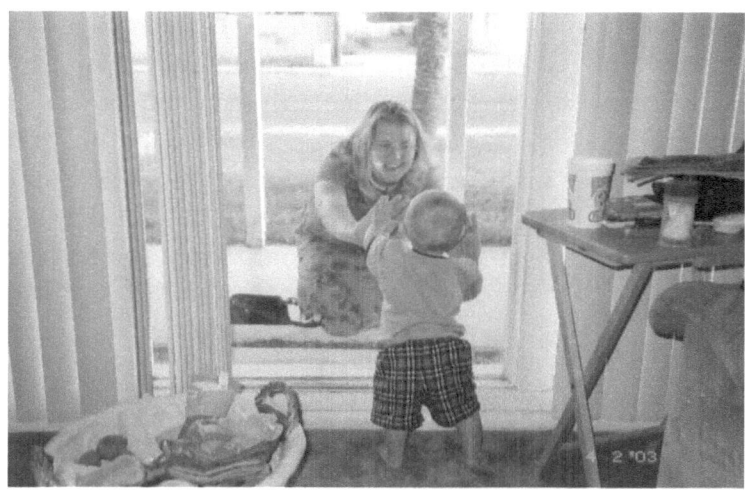

April 8: I've been noticing for a few weeks that Jake's skin on his knees is getting rougher, from rug burn. He's always crawling around. I hate for any of his soft skin to change! Today I realized that the tops of his feet are really sore from rug burn, so I rubbed massage oil on them today. They feel rough like eczema.

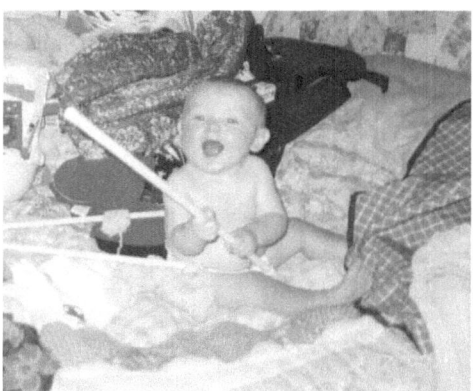

April 10: Today is my 33½ half-birthday. And today Jake was fussy for the first time as I left for work. He was standing at Grandma's screen door, watching me and said "MA!" He says "muh-muh-muh" a lot,

but we're not convinced it means anything. I've been taking him over to Grandma and Gramps' house just about every workday now, because it frees up some morning time for Grandma, lets me spend a few extra minutes with Jake and keeps Scott from being late to school. I love this extra time with Jake in the mornings as much as Scott enjoys spending the afternoons with him. He picks Jake up every day and they have playtime alone together for over an hour, before or after Jake's late afternoon nap.

April 12: Jake is just shy of 10 months old and today he stands alone for two seconds! Today we discuss selecting a guardian for Jake and writing our wills. It's such an important choice and so very difficult.

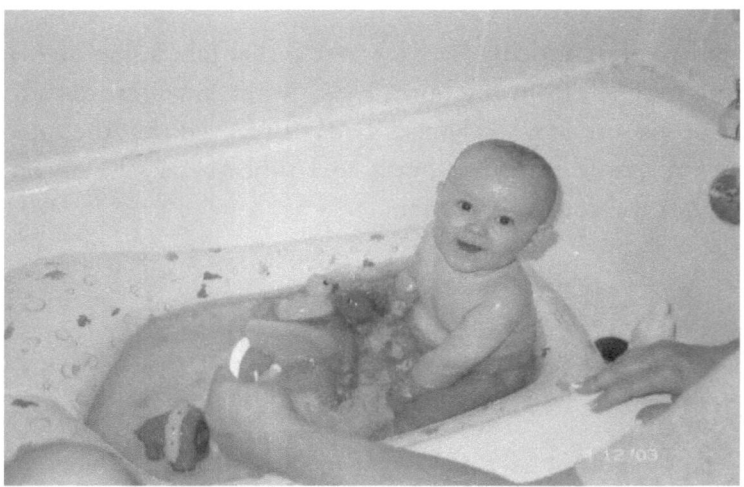

April 15: Jake at 10 months old:

- He's 22 lbs, with clothes on, (size 4 Pampers) and 28¼ inches. He wears 12-18 month clothes.

- He eats small bites of solid food now; loves Cheerios and raisins.

- We continue to spoonfeed applesauce and our leftover Stage 2 & 3 baby food.

- He drinks 12-20 oz of formula per day, usually in the form of "sleepy bottles", which contain the "magic sleeping potion."

- He still naps 1½ hours in the late morning and up to an hour in the late afternoon.

- Nighttime: often sleeps 10 hours straight! (9:30 p.m.-7:30 a.m.)

- He crawls fast, investigates, stands by furniture and is beginning to test his balance for a few seconds. Due to his ability to stand, we've moved his crib mattress down to the lowest of 3 levels.

- He's very happy, smiley, giggly and playful. He holds onto a ball, climbs on Daddy, looks in the mirror, and flips upside down with Mama.

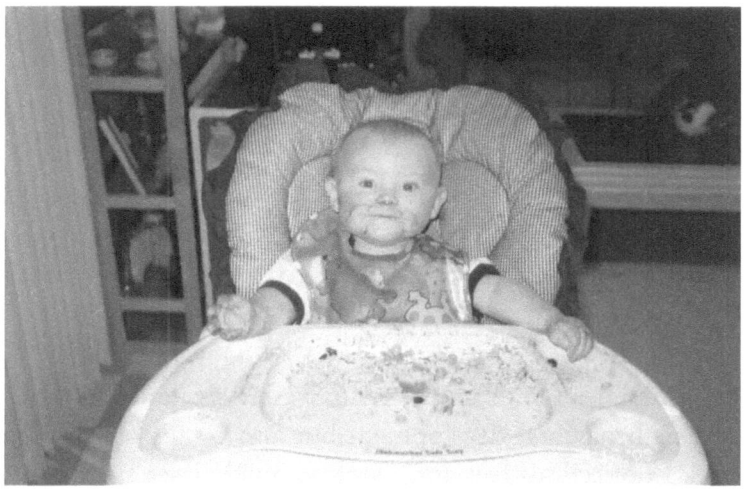

April 25: Jake stands alone now for up to five seconds!

April 29: He has started learning about waving and he's definitely "cruising" around furniture now!

May 2: Jake is 10½ months now! Grandma brings Jake on a field trip to Mama's office! After touring the assembly area in the plant, he waves bye-bye in return to some of the ladies! This is the first time he does it in response to someone else waving, with no coaching from us.

May 7: Jake is now crawling from room to room, exploring as he goes! And what is incredible to me is that he actually remembers where he left off the last time he was in that room and goes straight back to it! He can entertain himself for 20-30 minutes, checking things out around the house. Nothing is off limits now and we have taken to shutting doors....

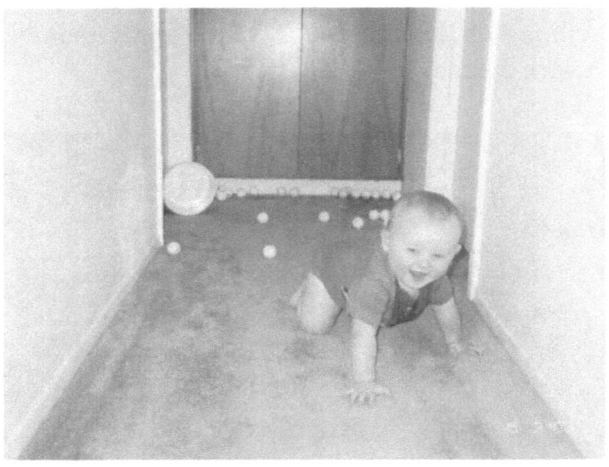

May 8: Sometimes I look at Jake "with fresh eyes" and I'm shocked by not only his behavioral development but also by his physical growth. This week I noticed his feet don't look so much like a baby's anymore, but more like those of a little boy. This makes me feel sad. As he approaches 11 months old, Jake's sleep schedule remains the same:

- Nighttime: 10½ hours is now optimal; usually sleeps straight through from 8:30 p.m. to around 7 a.m.

- Morning nap: approx 10:30-noon

- Afternoon nap: 3:30-4:30, usually falling asleep in Daddy's Jeep

May 9: Today is Friday and I take an official "vacation day" to stay with Jake. How fun! I don't do a single thing that is work-related. It's very rare when I'm home to not even check my e-mail, ingrained during the Fridays when I was "working from home" and always "on call" for questions and emergencies like rush wire transfer prepayments to new vendors or some such thing. After we have breakfast, we run errands, delivering Daddy some flowers for Teacher Appreciation Week and then we meet Alisa, Lauren and Kayden for lunch at Chandler Fashion Center. For my first Mother's Day gift, Jake buys me Theo Huxtable Eggen Bear from Build-a-Bear!…Jake loves birdies, airplanes and rocks. He still loves exploring and is now learning how to "throw" (give) a ball. He seems slightly less interested in *Teletubbies* these days, but really likes Big Bird and Elmo. He also loves to watch *The Wiggles* and his cherished *Baby Einstein* videos.

May 11: Today is my very first Mother's Day! I love that little boy! It's so fun to give him his nighttime "sleepy bottle" at around 9 p.m. He just crashes by the end of it and I love feeling him asleep nestled in the crook of my left elbow. He is my precious angel baby.

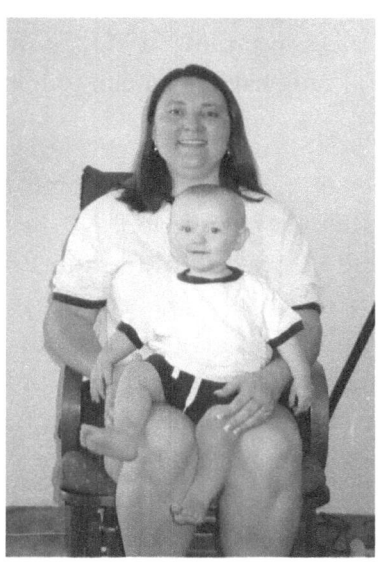

May 12: I've noticed how he is beginning to wrap himself around us now when he's being picked up. He holds on to our shirt with his little hands and curls his legs a little around our waist. Grandma reports that he has been quite "vocal" today, telling her what he wants!

May 13: Tonight Jake has his first dinner at Macayo's in a high chair and he even orders a hamburger off the kids' menu! It was strange because our server, a male, called Jake "an angel". Jake is about two days away from finishing off an entire box of Cheerios all by himself.

May 14: For nearly a month, Jake has been fidgety when I change him, trying to turn over and even getting up on his knees! Well, now he's trying to pull this funny business with his daddy and his grandma also so I'm not "the only one"! He fusses and fusses when we change his diaper. He didn't used to be like this. Sometimes we can use a diversion like a book or toy to get through a diaper change.

May 15: The little guy is 11 months old! He can now "throw" a ball to us, at a maximum distance of about 12 inches. It's very cute. He loves squishy ones, like his orange "basketball" and his Sesame Street "soccer ball", both of which have a 4-5" diameter. Tonight, for the very first time in his life, Jake falls asleep ON HIS OWN in his crib, after refusing his bottle. In fact, I only have to go talk to him once.

May 19: This book project is a slow mover. In our fast-paced world, it's a snail. After postponing the "book release" nearly nine months, I've set myself a schedule for completion. No goal, no getting it done. Aunt Heidi baked while I typed for three hours straight. Deception is absolutely necessary at this point.... Jake is adorable when he is investigating and concentrating. He says "puh, puh, puh" or "doo" and "doe". We have to keep his "paci" in his mouth when he's playing in our room because many small things are magnets for his attention: especially my chapstick on the bedstand and the rocks in the fountain. He loves the skein of yarn I bought years ago, along with a training book *How to Knit*, which remains unopened.

May 20: Jake continues to require 13 hours of sleep per day, total. And, regardless of what is published on the topic of weaning from a bottle, he continues to greatly enjoy sucking. I don't expect to attempt to wean him from his bottle until he is 15-18 months, at least. When he needs his "night-night" bottle, he has actually picked up his paci and inserted it into his mouth! His other signs that he's tired: yawning, rubbing his eyes with his blankie or the closest available object including the remote control or my chest, lying on the floor face down in the blankie for a few seconds.... Jake is very deliberate in his actions and learns quickly from his "mistakes" or missteps. His feelings are quite transparent.... He's never wanted to venture into the yard before, but today he decided he was ready and sat on the grass near the front patio. All of a sudden he crawled like lightning across our unfenced front yard, toward Old Colony. I was amused, but was watching him carefully and as I stepped from behind our tree to gather him up before he got too close to the sidewalk, I see a woman running towards him, with her van stopped at the stop sign and the door open! It took us each a few seconds to realize what was happening and that we had each been invisible to each other. It was this Good Samaritan who had gotten Jake's attention and he wanted to go say hi to her! Later in the day we walked through the neighborhood until I spotted her van and thanked her properly for her concern for my sweet baby. Not everyone would have stopped.... Jake eats small bites of whatever we are eating now, in addition to a few Cheerios. He has a "sleepy bottle" before naps and bedtime, and occasionally an afternoon bottle. He is averaging 12-15 oz of formula a day. We can start feeding him whole milk in three weeks! A 4-oz serving of formula costs $.50, so milk will really seem like a bargain (a box containing 18 individual serving packets costs $9; we do keep a $12 can on hand, with a scoop for every 2 oz, which is convenient since he often drinks a 6-oz bottle).

May 26: We spend three days in DeKalb and Chicago, celebrating Auntie Stephanie's graduation from Northern Illinois University College of Law! We have so much fun on this trip and Jake is a great traveler. The DeKalb Best Western provides us with a crib and this works out great. At 11¼ months, Jake now waves bye-bye on demand, or of his own free will.

May 27: Jake allows me to rock him for 20 minutes, from 5:20-5:40 a.m. This is a very special and rare treat for me.

May 28: Jake waves bye-bye spontaneously to the *Teletubbies*. He is madly in love with *Baby Dolittle*. He screeches and bounces in his saucer.

May 30: Jake is no longer the baby in the extended family: Emersyn Paige is born this evening at the same hospital. Holly and new baby (#4) are doing well.

June 1: Jake is now 11½ months old. This past week he started very cautiously taking 1-2 steps alone. He's very careful and determined.... I love giving Jake his "sleepy bottle" at night. This is usually my job, since Scott is often on-line updating his website, watching the news or reading headline articles on AOL! Since Scott is on "baby duty" from 3:15-6:30 p.m., this time after we eat dinner and play is often his first few minutes he has to himself all day. Anyway, as he drinks his bottle, Jake touches the edge of his blankie over and over. He holds it between his thumb and forefinger. Finally he relaxes, eventually slowing and then stopping his sucking completely, snuggled, sweaty, in the crook of my left elbow. I often nod off, too. It's very snuggly. Then I lay him carefully in his crib. This doesn't wake him; then he likes to roll over onto his left side. He's out for ten hours!

June 2: Today is Jake's last full day with Grandma before summer vacation with Daddy! They end up spending three hours in the pool under the canopied pool lounge seat. It's Jake first swim of the season.

June 5: In celebration of Grandpa's 62nd birthday, Jake takes 4-5 steps, unassisted, before plopping down or grabbing onto furniture. In their first week of vacation together, Scott is having so much fun with Jake. I take Jake on a baby modeling audition today and we pick up Grandpa from work for a special birthday lunch.

June 6: News in Jakeland at 11 2/3 months!

- He points at objects or at anything he wants to tell us about: airplanes, lights, how Daddy's behind the bathroom door.

- He self-feeds very well and eats anything, until he's full, at which point he stops abruptly. He ate an entire sliced banana last night, but is losing interest in the Graduates ravioli.

- He does not like to hold his own juice cup or bottle yet.

- He often takes 3-5 steps unassisted.

- He loves windchimes (has even played two at a time, one with each hand), birdies, balls, airplanes, lights and Baby Einstein videos.

June 7: Jake's first time in a lake: Canyon Lake with Daddy, Mama, Grandma, Gramps, Aunt Heidi and Uncle Bill. We are there together from 11:40 a.m. to 4:30 p.m.

June 8: Jake loves Mama's yarn and drags it through the house! I now have my own office, with four walls and a door, and Jake and Grandma accompany me there today (Sunday) to continue unpacking. Afterwards Heidi meets us for lunch at Arizona Mills mall. Jake has Panda Express Orange Chicken for the first time and Mama buys him a Pooh balloon, which he loves. At the mall we lose the "extra" sleepy-blankie, so we are down to one. When we go over to Aunt Heidi's later, Jake is very active and climbs the entire staircase 5 or 6 times! What an adventure! I realize that, (surprise!), Jake has a molar coming in—bottom left gum…. Tonight Jake experiences his first bad fall: he is playing on the guest bed, with Mama right there folding laundry, and, partially due to the water tube mattress' instability, Jake flops over the side, hitting the wall and lodging himself between the bed frame and the wall. Mama screams for Daddy and he and Uncle Sean come running. Jake is very sad after we retrieve him, and a nice bruised bump on his forehead asserts itself. Daddy says it's better to have a bump than not to have a bump.

June 9: Daddy reports that Jake walks a distance of SIX FEET today!

June 11: Grandma and Mama help Jake make handprints on a Father's Day shirt for Daddy. His blue fingernails are a dead giveaway!

June 12: Jake is becoming a confident walker already. He can go 10-12 feet with no problem. In fact, this evening, with Daddy out back grilling chicken, he steps right out the back door! He often will push a door open now, if it's ajar, and even moves the baby gate aside if we don't have it locked in place!…The baby modeling agency where we auditioned last week responded by saying Jake is "very cute" and they are "definitely interested" in him, but expect us to dish out $545 for marketing photos with no guarantee of a future paying job. We've made the decision not to do it because of the slight possibility of not recouping our investment. Even though the BBB rates this place as "satisfactory", you never know what kind of operation they are running.… Today Jake and Scott visit me at my new office! Yes, it's a little dreary and claustrophobic to have no windows, but I do love having my own room. Even with the door open, it's really quiet and I'm able to just sit and work and mind my own business. After working in a cubicle for 10 years, what a change this is. Plus I have three plants and a bouquet of fresh flowers!…Jake nestles and falls asleep in just five minutes with his sleepy bottle tonight. I love this time.

Part III:
One Year Old!

✦

(already)

From: Elaine
Sent: Friday, June 13, 2003 5:19 PM
To: Monica; scooter; heidip

Sunday is the day of all days since the foundation of the earth. I think it's referred to in Revelations—do you remember?? "Harken to these words: Life shall come to a sudden halt when the small boy Jake completes his first year. Parents, friends, those with common blood and acquaintances will journey from the ends of the hot place to honor the child. All manner of tributes will be placed at his feet, and he shall run down the hall pointing and shouting "UH." All who care will feast and look on with amazement."

June 14: Wow. This will be the only time I am actually typing directly into this document on the very day it is happening. This is it. The culmination of the first year of Jake's life. Tomorrow we will be celebrating among many, many friends and family. In fact, our party RSVPs indicate we will have 24 adults plus 10 kids! We've rented 10 extra chairs, picked up the strawberry banana cream cake from Cathy's Rum Cake Caterers and we'll be making the ice cream mix tonight! Safeway has donated a free cake to the cause as well, which we may let Jake play in. It's strange to think how this time last year we were spending the evening at Mom's, placing bets on when the delivery date might be. And little did we know my water would break less than 12 hours after that! I felt so big and uncomfortable. But of course it's all worth it. I'd do it all over again…and again. Jake will be a great big brother someday. And every one of his brothers and sisters deserves a book, too, but they probably won't get one. They'll get something else in their name, though. And they'll get an awesome big brother.

Oh, Jake just woke up from a much-needed nap, following his one-year portrait session at Sears. I think he has something to add to this document. Here he goes at the keyboard!

Nnnnnnnnnnnm., 0063zA

(Jake typed that)

Some things we'll always want to remember about Jake at this age:

- His singing and humming when wandering around by himself.
- His first time walking into our shower and plopping down.
- How he firmly points at his bedroom lamp first thing in the morning so you know he wants you to turn it on…*NOW!*
- How much he wants to talk and tell us what he's thinking about!
- How he first took my hand as we walked next door together.
- How he loves the American flag, airplanes and balls—how his face just lights up and how brightly he smiles!
- How he pops his paci into his mouth whenever he decides he needs it.
- How he comes a-runnin' whenever I flush the toilet, so he can watch the water go down and try to stick his hand in the bowl before Mama grabs it!
- How he wants to eat rocks and gets mad when I take them away from him.
- How he giggles when Daddy says, "I'm gonna get ya!"
- How he giggles when we're riding in the car and I copy his shrieks and "ma-ma-ma-ma"s.
- How cute the dimples in his elbows are!
- How he'll be so excited when I finish typing this book so I can get up from the computer desk and play with him!

June 15, 2003: Today Jake turns 1 and Scott gets his 2nd Father's Day! Jake was such a nice Father's Day gift last year! For Father's Day, Jake gets Daddy socks, briefs, a pair of boxers and the *Jungle Book 2* DVD. From me, Scott receives 2 books, a King Louie stuffed animal and, presented later, a DVD/VCR combo. (Hey, I had to compete with the Xbox precedent I'd set last year!) For Jake's First Birthday breakfast, he has Cheerios, cheese bites, Gerber Graduates chicken sticks, ½ a slice of whole wheat bread, diced peaches and apple juice in a cup.... Jake hasn't nursed in 4 months or so, but I still have milk. I even leak a drop or two sometimes when he snuggles with his bottle.... We all survive Jake's first birthday celebration in good shape and although the poor child goes six straight hours without a nap, he really does well. He is very excited about the balloons Grandma brings; he smears the cake icing in his face and there's pretty much a food coloring overdose on his body; then he tastes the icing and doesn't even eat a bit of cake. Primary colors all mixed together really make an ugly shade of dark green. All of Jake's 31 guests enjoy the catered cake and homemade vanilla ice cream, plus sherbet lemonade punch. Then we cram everyone into the great room as he watches his parents open all the toys, books and clothes a one-year-old could ever want or need. He's very interested in his Fisher-Price zoo (of which he is now the proud owner of 2 complete sets) and his new learning toy with lights. Also of interest are various stuffed animals. But his favorite gifts are from Daddy: two small American flags he can wave around. He's very patriotic, at least by appearances. Mama presents him with a Buzz Lightyear bubble machine (but no batteries), an Elmo night-night book in preparation for bottle weaning and Kaa, to maintain the *Jungle Book* theme of the day. Daddy selected several more *Baby Einstein* videos which are a guaranteed hit. Just when we think his "sleepy bottle" might help him drift off for a much needed nap, he sits up and starts walking around again, to Grandma's great disappointment. Then Mama puts him in his new floaty swimsuit and we join the six kids and two parents already in the pool. Jake looks like royalty in his canopied floating seat, much like a small Indian prince sitting in a gazebo on the back of an elephant. Daddy grills and grills. For his birthday dinner, Jake has a few bites of cheeseburger with lettuce and tomato, accompanied by ranch beans, watermelon, potato salad and Cheerios. He and his Uncles Duane and Doug have a clapping tournament following dinner. Then the one-year-old baby gently falls sound asleep in the back of

Daddy's Jeep on the way to Tempe Sports Complex, where his parents try to scrape up enough energy to play coed softball.

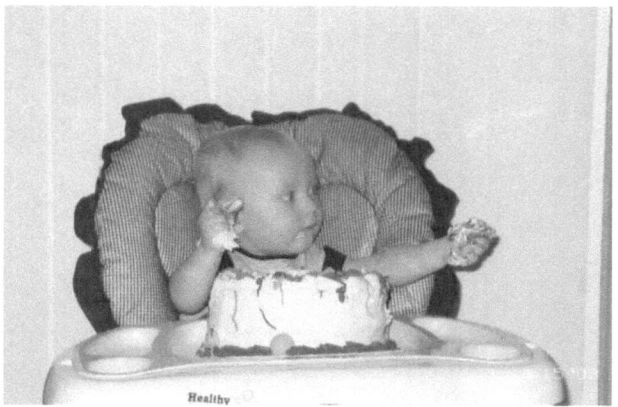

Epilogue

Don't worry about a thing
'Cause every little thing's gonna be alright
This is my message to you....

Bob Marley's got the right idea. We can't predict the future, but we can just do our best to prepare for it, and prepare our little ones for it. They are truly our future and we've seen that it really does take a village to raise a child. We sincerely value the time and efforts made by various members of our families with respect to Jake's care. As Graham Nash wrote for Crosby Stills Nash & Young nearly 30 years ago, "teach your children well...." It would do us all well to remember:

> *If children live with criticism,*
> > *They learn to condemn.*
> *If children live with hostility,*
> > *They learn to fight.*
> *If children live with tolerance,*
> > *They learn to be patient.*
> *If children live with acceptance,*
> > *They learn to love.*
> *If children live with security,*
> > *They learn to have faith in themselves and others.*
> *If children live with friendliness,*
> > *They learn the world is a nice place in which to live.*

—excerpted from Dorothy Law Nolte, PhD

Someday, if we're lucky, we'll have more little ones running around the house, and maybe it'll even be a different house. Who knows. One day at a time.

We love you so very much, Jake. And even though we don't know your name(s) yet, we love you so very much, Jake's future younger brother(s) or sister(s). Thank you all for adding much joy to our lives.

Thank you, Husband, for being both an excellent person and an excellent father to our children. I never could have imagined this wonderful, crazy life. Team Eggen is so much fun!

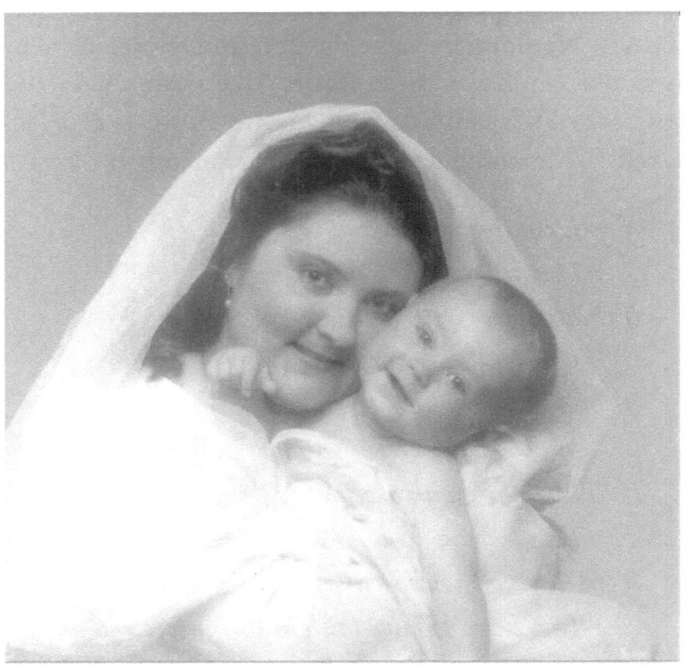

Acknowledgements

The author is eternally grateful to William and Heidi Thomas for their willing assistance during the last few months of this project. I couldn't have finished in any sort of timely, or untimely, manner, were it not for your time, energy and slyness. Thanks to Bill for the many tedious hours he spent editing and to Heidi for baking and babysitting the sweet baby doll. Anyone reading this can thank Bill for declaring this work suitable for public consumption. Scott, I can only say that you greatly *"underestimated our sneakiness"* and I sure do hope that you didn't see this file in My Documents.

"Thank you" isn't enough to properly acknowledge Alisa Yocum and Elaine Miller for providing Jake with a loving, enriching environment. We so appreciate what you've done for Jake during the weekdays when our work keeps us from our precious baby boy.

The Discovery Channel/TLC's wonderful television stories including "A Baby Story", "A Wedding Story" and "A Dating Story" helped provide the inspiration for this autobiographical effort and the author would like to recognize the producers of such excellent true-to-life programming.

The author would also like to express a heartfelt thank you to Vicki Iovine for writing and publishing *The Girlfriends' Guide to Pregnancy* and *The Girlfriends' Guide to Surviving The First Year of Motherhood*. These words got me through the rough postpartum months when I wondered if I would ever get a full night's sleep again. Ms. Iovine's advice instilled hope in an exhausted new mother. Where this book may be honest, her books are both honest *and* witty.

Julie Aigner-Clark also deserves a big "high five" for her genius in creating the *Baby Einstein* series of videos. These alone allow us up to 29 minutes to read the mail, eat breakfast, shower, return a phone call or...type a paragraph. Jake squeals, points, smiles and grunts at the toys and animals, but doesn't take his eyes off the screen. They are truly excellent materials and Jake loves them dearly.